African Studies

History, Politics, Economics, Culture

Edited by

Molefi Asante
Temple University

A Routledge Series

African Studies
History, Politics, Economics, Culture
Molefi Asante, *General Editor*

Kwame Nkrumah's Contribution to
Pan-Africanism
An Afrocentric Analysis
D. Zizwe Poe

Nyansapo (The Wisdom Knot)
Toward an African Philosophy of Education
Kwadwo A. Okrah

The Yorùbá Traditional Healers of Nigeria

Mary Olufunmilayo Adekson

Routledge
Taylor & Francis Group
NEW YORK AND LONDON

Published in 2003 by
Routledge
711 Third Avenue,
New York, NY 10017
www.routledge-ny.com

Published in Great Britain by
Routledge
2 Park Square, Milton Park,
Abingdon, Oxon, OX14 4RN
www.routledge.co.uk

Routledge is an imprint of the Taylor & Francis Group

Transferred to Digital Printing 2005

First issued in paperback 2012

ISBN 13: 978-0-415-65481-4 (pbk)
ISBN 13: 978-0-415-94580-6 (hbk)

Library of Congress Cataloging-in-Publication Data

Adekson, Mary Olufunmilayo
The Yorùbá traditional healers of Nigeria / by Mary Olufunmilayo Adekson.
p. cm. — (African studies)
Includes bibliographical references (p.).
ISBN 0-415-94580-1
1. Yoruba (African people)—Medicine. 2. Healers—Nigeria. 3. Counseling—Nigeria.
I. Title. II. Series: African studies (Routledge (Firm)).
DT515.45.Y67A226 2003
615.8'8'089963330669—dc21 2003007179

To my two wonderful children,
Adedayo Oluwakayode and Babatunde Oluwaseun

Contents

Foreword

DURING THE LAST TWENTY-FIVE YEARS, I HAVE MADE SIX TRIPS TO AFRICA TO interview traditional healers and their patients. I use the word *healer* instead of doctor to refer to holistic lay practitioners who treat more than eighty percent of the people in sub-Saharan Africa. Serving concurrently as psychologist, sociologist, physician, spiritual leader, and magician, they treat all problems since specialists are generally unavailable. In rare cases where another generalist is within walking distance, a healer may specialize in setting bones or "fixing" minds. I use the phrase *traditional healer* to differentiate them from physicians, psychologists, social workers, counselors, and other healthcare personnel trained in Western methods of healing. Although Western-style professionals are found in large cities in Africa, few people can afford to pay their consultation fee or buy the medicine they prescribe.

There are several differences between American counseling and its equivalent in traditional Africa. How people are screened into the helping profession represents an important distinction. In the United States, counseling usually requires the use of standardized tests and "well conceived theories." It is generally considered a science rather than an art. One justification for this assertion is the manner in which applicants for admission to counselor training programs in graduate schools are screened. In general, they are required to take the Graduate Record Examination or some other empirically-tested, "valid" and "reliable" psychometric instrument. For the most part, only academically-qualified students are admitted to counselor education programs.

In traditional Africa, many healers declare that they were "called." Evidence of the calling can be spotted in children as young as five. In visiting a family in Ivory Coast, I talked with the mother of a six-year old boy who indicated that her son was going to be a healer like his grandfather, because the child reflected the sagacity of his departed ancestor. Members of the family respected the little boy's judgment so much that they consulted him before they made important decisions. Once such an individual is "spotted," he (the person is usually a male) may be apprenticed to a healer for up to fifteen or twenty years, during which time he learns a great deal about human nature, healing properties of plants, bark, and roots, and therapeutic rituals.

In the United States, psychological theory is an important part of most counselor education programs. In traditional Africa, a codified healing theory does not exist. Instead, there exists a philosophy of nature that holds that everything in the universe is a single living, breathing, and responsive organism. Therefore, all of nature is connected. If a healer wants to diagnose a problem or malady in a human being, it may be reasonable and insightful to study the direction in which caged mice run or to observe the configuration of thrown cow chips on the ground. "Reading" the direction of running mice and the spread of chips are just two of the many procedures used by healers to determine what is wrong with their clients.

Conversely, American counselors depend on scientifically-validated instruments, research, and therapeutic procedures. Over the last forty years, school-related "helping" evolved from guidance to counseling, which today is not easily distinguishable from psychotherapy. In the 1950s and 1960s, many school principals selected teachers who demonstrated a special ability to relate to children and assigned them counseling duties, even when they lacked professional training as a counselor. Today, counselor educators and employers usually consider academic acumen and scientific knowledge to be more important than "people skills," which, although desirable, can not be empirically measured. Students who have nothing to offer but relationship skills usually do not get through graduate school.

On the other hand, in traditional Africa, the most important quality that healers exhibit is their authority and healing charisma; traits that are usually personified in old people. Throughout my years of travel in Africa, I have never met a healer younger than fifty years. However, in the United States, psychotherapeutic knowledge can be obtained by anyone who is intelligent enough to read university textbooks, use the library, surf the internet, and pass courses required for graduation, licensure, or certification purposes. Once they receive the stamp of approval from whatever governmental body to which they must present their credentials, they are among the helpers foreign-born persons consult for direction and assistance. Unfortunately, many culturally-different clients from traditional societies are unable to relate to our scientist-counselors, because such people are external to their understanding of helping and the person of the helper.

Another important difference between American-style counseling and traditional African healing is client participation. In the U. S., the prevalent therapeutic model requires that clients provide continuous verbal and nonverbal content that counselors interpret. The practice is based on the belief that therapeutic interpretation triggers insight that, in turn, enhances mental health and desired social behavior. In traditional Africa, the helper is an authority figure who prescribes therapeutic remedies and objects designed to eradicate human problems. In some cases, clients do not engage in a therapeutic dialogue. They may not even state the presenting problem. The head of the family may be the one who describes the symptoms of the relative needing treatment.

Helping cannot be divorced from the culture in which individuals and their problems in life develop and reside. A culturally-symbiotic relationship exists between the counselor and client. Counselors are most effective helping their cultural peers who are products of the same socialization as they are. Their counseling competency is put to test by clients from non-Western countries who consulted traditional healers back home. In order to benefit such clients, they need to acquire as much information as possible about the kind of helping their culturally-different clients received in their native country. They may even try to incorporate some of the traditional African healing techniques in their work with immigrant clients.

Professor Mary Adekson's book adds to the growing body of literature on traditional healing in Africa. Scientifically trained American and European counselors need not abandon their usual approaches to therapy. With the information provided in this book, they can decide what aspects of traditional healing they want to consider using in helping all clients, not just those from developing countries in which most people depend on healers such as the ones described by Dr. Adekson. American psychotherapeutic professionals must be open to learning from traditional healers, as they are open to learning from us.

Clemmont E. Vontress, PhD
Professor Emeritus of Counseling
George Washington University.

Acknowledgements

I am grateful to God for giving me the wisdom to finish this book. To God be the glory great things He hath done. And He said the things which are impossible with men are possible with God (Luke 18:27) but with God all things are possible (Mathew 19: 26). Great is the Lord's doing, it is marvelous in our eyes! Ohun ti Jesu ati Eleda mi se IYANU lo je. I owe the preservation of my life, my childrens' and my family to God for giving us the endurance, perseverance and long life to start and finish this book. May all the glory go to Him. Amen.

I am grateful to Drs. Richard Hazler, Tom Davis, Thomas Sweeney and Lisa Lopez Levers for suggesting that I undertake this research on The Yorùbá Traditional Healers.

I also cherish the support and advice of Dr. Jake Johnson, Dr. M. Gyi, Professors Clemmont Vontress, M. Akin Mákindé, Akínṣọlá Akìwọwọ and Olú Mákindé, Mrs. Tokunbo Adekambi and family, Dr. Demola Ariyo, Dr. Milton Ploghoft, Dr. Larry and Mary Jageman, Kunle Lawal, James Finch (my technical adviser), Dr. Carol Anne Pierson, former Dean of the College of Education at St. Bonaventure University, Andrea Puls, Theresa Shaffer, Kimberly Jackson, Merrilee White, Dr. Eleanor English, Dr. Paul Schafer, Dr. Reba Powers, Taresa Carro, Betty Lyman and Mary Monterville. I am also grateful for the assistance of my children, parents Pa G.O. Williams and Chief Mrs. D.A. Williams, brothers, Mofoluwaṣọ, Olanrewaju and Agboọla and sisters, Moṣebọlatan and Olajumọkẹ.

I also wish to acknowledge the assistance, cooperation, fatherly love, sincerity, and honesty of Chief Awórẹni, The *Àràbà* of *Ilé-Ifẹ̀* and the *Oníṣẹ̀sìn Àgbáyé*, Chief Awójọbí, Chief Ọlájídé and Dr. E. A. Awótáyò, Dr. (Alhaji) Akinọlá, Chief James Abíọ́lá and Dr. Adéoyè Adésànyà, the Yoruba Traditional Healers interviewed and videotaped for this book. May God Bless and give you long life and wisdom to continue to assist clients towards holistic health Amen.

Lastly, I wish to express my gratitude to Professor Molefi Asante of Temple University, Kimberly Guinta, and John Shea of Routledge Publishing Company and Farideh Kamali former Dissertation Editor at Routledge.

CHAPTER ONE

Introduction

Cultural and Methodological Context

Most of the existing studies on traditional healers in Africa were conducted by Western anthropologists, sociologists, psychologists, and psychiatrists. Researchers such as Margaret Mead, Jahoda (1961), Kahn and Delk (1973), Kramer (1970), and Kelly (1965) elicited vital information by living with so-called "natives" in different cultures in the developing world. Information derived from these studies has contributed to the field of psychotherapy, even though Western scientists view traditional healing systems, such as those prevalent in Africa, as primitive and non-therapeutic (Ìdòwú, 1985).

Research conducted by Western researchers, though important, lacks the richness and depth available from scholars of non-Western cultures. According to Ahia and Bradley (1984), most researchers in this category are affluent, well-meaning and adventurous Westerners like Drewal (1992) who are not representatives of the culture under investigation. Mákindé (1988) further contended that major debates on African culture over the past two hundred years have been conducted by Europeans for Europeans.

Consequently, "if we are to truly begin to talk to Africans and not just about them, we need to hear the African side of the story from the African point of view" (Mákindé, 1988, p.xxi). Since culture has a potentially great impact on the counseling relationship and its outcome, studies done by researchers from the same culture elicit information that is richer and more eye-opening (Saleh, 1989).

Traditional healers have unique roles to play in psychotherapy and medicine, both in Africa and in the rest of the world. The uniqueness of Africa as a continent with its rich cultural heritage and people therefore supports the usefulness of and need for this study. Equally, Torrey (1986) argued that,

> regardless of what one believes about the desirability of promoting or not promoting the use of indigenous therapists in third world cultures, the fact remains that such therapists are today the only psychotherapeutic (and often medical) resource for the majority of the world's population (p. 185).

A triadic or three-pronged counseling relationship exists between a counselor, client, and a third party culture (Saleh, 1989). In this vein, this volume analyzed the functions performed and interpersonal techniques used by seven Yorùbá Traditional Healers of South-Western Nigeria. The author specifically examined the culture of these healers and observed their interactions with clients during individual and group divining sessions through observations of videotaped live sessions and interviews in *Yorùbá* land. However, due to time constraints, only five (four herbalists and one diviner) healers were interviewed.

It is hoped that this study, which was conducted in 1994, will contribute to the literature on these healers because the researcher is a *Yorùbá* woman who holds the same fundamental beliefs about, and comes from the same culture as, the traditional healers. It is also hoped that this volume, which provides interesting facts on healers' physical, interpersonal and personal or private worlds (Binswanger, 1962), will help readers gain a deeper understanding of healers' "everyday experiences" (van Manen, 1990).

METHODOLOGY AND HYPOTHESES

The volume employed an exploratory case study method and incorporated the participant observation method in the investigation of the roles, functions and services of, and the interpersonal techniques used by, Yorùbá Traditional Healers (YTH). This method is supported by Frey (1978), Ary, Jacobs, and Razavich (1979), Kazdin (1980), Merriam (1988), and Yin (1994). Yin (1994) referred to a case study as "an empirical inquiry that investigates a contemporary phenomenon within its real life context" (p.13), especially when the boundaries between phenomenon and context are not clearly evident. Chassan (1967) also maintained that case studies allow in-depth examination of group research, while Goldman (1978) and Frey (1978) argued that they enable the researcher to probe issues in an intensive, in-depth and holistic manner.

The case study is typically an inductive research method, which does not postulate or test hypotheses but generates them (Van Dalen & Meyer, 1966). According to Frey (1978), hypotheses are not developed from case research until the data collection process has been completed. Yin (1994) added that the goal of case study is to "develop pertinent hypotheses and propositions for further inquiry" (p.5) and Merriam (1988) confirmed that the case study has been widely used "to build theories when there is none available to explain a particular phenomenon" (p.59).

Furthermore, Kazdin (1980) asserted that the case study, as used in psychological research, has provided theories about the etiology of psychological disorder, produced theories about behavior in general and has been advanced by the impetus behind the study of individual cases. "The case study, like other research strategies, is a way of investigating an empirical topic by following a set of pre-specified procedures" (Yin, 1994, p. 15).

The inductive nature of the case study research provides the investigator with a better understanding of various and basic aspects of human behavior (Ary, Jacobs, & Razavich, 1979, Johnson, 1986). It also offers the researcher an "intensive probing" technique which may assist in revealing unanticipated information about "relationships" (Ary, Jacobs, & Razavich, 1979). Miller and Warner (1975) agreed that the case study not only provides for the collection of extensive data regarding a client's or individual's behavior in general, it also provides other data on him or her relating to "health, socio-economic status" and much more.

In Chapters Four and Five, this volume formulated hypotheses that attempt to explain the interpersonal techniques used by Yorùbá Traditional Healers. Moreover, this study analyzes healers' communication patterns, functions, daily activities, interactional relationships, categories of behavior and services. The hypotheses developed from this study explained how Yorùbá Traditional Healers impacted the interpersonal world of the persons (clients) under investigation (Binswanger, 1962, 1963).

In order to improve objectivity, triangulation, which is the use of "multiple sources of evidence" such as participant observation, interview schedules and physical evidence, like videotaping (Yin, 1984,1994), was used to collect data on Yorùbá Traditional Healers. I observed, interviewed, videotaped and kept journals on each healer. Interview schedule, which is a set of questions administered to all respondents/healers (Appendix B & C), provided standardization and structure, and permitted the respondent to amplify and or qualify needed responses (Johnson, 1986). Records of Yorùbá Traditional Healers' thoughts, behaviors, as well as verbal and non-verbal interactions were also kept by the investigator. Additional information was obtained through participant observation and journals to supplement the case facts derived from the use of an interview schedule.

Need for the Study

The present volume is important for several reasons. Firstly, there is a pressing need to understand the interpersonal techniques used by Yorùbá Traditional Healers of Nigeria, since each human being exists in a unique physical, interpersonal, and private world (Binswanger,1962). As such, the Yorùbá Traditional Healers' interpersonal relationships necessarily affect their communication patterns with their clients.

Secondly, due to the dearth of data on interpersonal techniques used by and the general activities of Yorùbá Traditional Healers, there is a need to fill the void in the literature. The World Health Organization (W.H.O.) (1977) suggested a need for more research to be undertaken on all aspects of traditional medicine (and healing or counseling, as it applies in this study) and to improve methods, techniques, and the composition of traditional medicaments. W.H.O. believes that there is a need to communicate such knowledge to political decision-makers and professional personnel employing other systems of medicine (or psychotherapy). Mákindé (1988) supported this need by concluding, "the world would be a better place to live in, if we come to know each other's way of life and thinking through proper integration" (p. xvi).

Thirdly, it is important to examine Yorùbá Traditional Healers' interactions and relationships with their clients in order to understand the healers' helping behaviors, roles, functions, techniques and services rendered within the *Yorùbá* cultural milieu. Such an understanding will help psychiatrists, psychologists, medical doctors, pharmacists, social workers, counselor educators, other helping professionals, administrators, and the World Health Organization (WHO) to learn more concerning the roles played by Traditional Healers. Mákindé (1988) stated that modern research and useful publications are the two avenues through which the secrecy and mystery surrounding African Traditional Healing can be unraveled.

Fourthly and relatedly, the observations derived from this study are designed to reduce these mysteries by building on the work of researchers such as Mákindé (1984), Mallum (1983), Mákindé (1988), Saleh (1989), and Ìpàye (1986). The Bethesda Maryland-based National Institutes of Health (NIH) showed support for W.H.O. directives in this regard when it opened a department of Alternative Medicine in January 1993 as mandated by the United States (U.S.) Congress in Washington, D.C. (Trachtman, 1994). Dr. Joe Jacobs, former head of the Alternative Medicine Department at NIH, invited personnel to research various types of alternative medicine in the United States and overseas (Trachtman, 1994).

Finally, the increased visibility given to Yorùbá Traditional Healers and their methods should add valuable knowledge to the field of psychotherapy by creating a better understanding of the factors that produce healing in non-Western cultures. This volume, therefore, supports the preceding goals by collecting and seeking information on the healing culture of Yorùbá Traditional Healers.

The results of this undertaking should assist counseling professors to determine which new techniques and practices could be incorporated into training Nigerian and African counselors, in addition to Western counseling theories currently being emphasized in Nigerian and other African universities. Saleh's point that "the direct transfer and adoption of counseling theories and approaches from one culture to another are highly suspect" (Saleh, 1989, p. 3) supports the potential value of this project. The insights derived from this volume will yield new hypotheses that should lead to the adoption of counseling theories useful for *Yorùbá* and African counselors, and their clients.

FOCUS AND POTENTIAL APPLICABILITY OF STUDY

Two basic assumptions were necessary to carry out the present study:

1. that all of the subjects would respond truthfully and openly to all questions of the interview.
2. that the investigator, being a *Yorùbá* female, would facilitate interpersonal rapport with the Yorùbá Traditional Healer male subjects.

The project studied only seven all-male traditional healers in *Yorùbá* land in the South-Western part of Nigeria. These Nigerian-born healers from the *Yorùbá* ethnic group resided in *Ọ̀yọ́*, *Ọ̀ṣun*, *Ògùn*, and *Ondó* States of Nigeria in 1994 and consisted of four herbalists and three diviners. Since *Yorùbá* healers have mostly been males, they usually have been referred to as *babalawo* (father of the secrets) and medicine man. Although this volume's choice of all-male Yorùbá Traditional Healers was made to ensure uniformity and consistency, this does not imply that female Yorùbá Traditional Healers are less efficient or effective. Yet, because the roles and functions of, and techniques used by, female Yorùbá Traditional Healers could be different because of gender, only their male counterparts were chosen.

Certain female traditional healers specialize as mediums, i.e. those who are endowed with the power to transmit messages from the dead to the living (Stoller, 1989). The *Yorùbá* and African female healers also specialize in treating hematological diseases, psychiatric disorders, polio, dental problems, gynecological issues, marital problems, infertility and other family crises (Makinde, 1974; Levers & Maki, 1994).

Not surprisingly, the results of this research may not have universal applicability because it utilized a case study approach that focused on Yorùbá Traditional Healers. Therefore, interpretation beyond that group of individuals can only be done in a tentative manner at this time. On a related note, this volume did not directly compare the techniques used by Nigerian Traditional Healers with Western counseling techniques. Instead, Traditional healing techniques were evaluated on their own merit without the bias of Western cultural involvement. In so doing, the findings that emerge from this study may not be directly comparable to Western theories, techniques, and research.

IMPORTANT/CRITICAL CONCEPTS, NAMES AND TERMS

The following words, concepts, names and terms, used throughout the volume, are defined specifically as follows:

Tradition

Tradition is the totality of socially-transmitted behavior patterns, arts, beliefs, institutions, and all other products of human work and thought characteristic of a community or population. Gould and Kolb (1964) described tradition as a neutral term used to denote the transmission, usually oral, activities, taste, or beliefs from one generation to the next.

Traditional Medicine

The term traditional medicine refers to the sum of all the knowledge and practices, whether explicable or not, used in diagnosis, prevention, and elimination of physical, mental, or social imbalance (W.H.O. Technical Reports, 1978, p. 23). Traditional medicine relies exclusively on practical experience and observation handed down from generation to generation, whether verbally or in writing (W.H.O. Technical Reports, 1978, p. 23).

The totality of what is known as traditional medicine among the *Yorùbá* consists of the practice of *Onísègùn/Adáhunṣe* (herbalists) and *Ifá priests* (diviners), with complementary roles (Mákindé, 1994). Herbalists have a broad knowledge of and prepare herbs needed for treatment. Diviners consult *Ifá* to discern the obstacles that may impede treatment.

Dr. Afọlábí Epega, a fifth generation *Yorùbá Ifá* priest (*babaláwo*) and Phillip Neimark, an American *babaláwo*, pointed out that diviners employ "the probabilities of future events by restoring harmonious balance in the individual through ritual, sacrifice, and prayer" (Epega & Neimark, 1995, p. viii). Epega & Neimark (1995) further observed that "the diviner sees what is likely to happen if clients remain in their current state and understand that restoring harmonious energy (through the right diagnosis with the divining chain) enables them to alter unpleasant future events" (p.viii), by focusing on the individuals and not on their problems.

Traditional Healers

Traditional healers specialize in healing different kinds of diseases and illnesses. Some specifically specialize in healing psychiatric problems, while others specialize in healing multifarious problems. For the purposes of this study, traditional healers are regarded as individuals who specialize in healing psychological, social, emotional, spiritual and holistic problems.

A review of the literature indicates that Africans, who have been trained in the western system of education, refer to traditional healers as native doctor or divinator (Mallum, 1983). They are also referred to as medicine-man, herbalist, witch-doctor, soothsayer, or seer by their clientele and the populace; and as sorcerer, magician, or occultist, depending on the function they perform at different times (Vontress, 1991).

Denga (1983) posited that traditional healers include: elders, diviners, soothsayers, priests, and magicians who are believed by some clients to possess supernatural powers and are thus capable of predicting and forecasting the fate of individuals. Traditional healers believe that a positive change can be effected in their clients through the use of a traditional directive approach (Mallum, 1983). Classified as men and women whose activities, fame, or prestige have culturally mythical explanations (Mallum, 1983), these traditional healers are usually associated with gods, religion, spirits, and supernatural powers.

Babaláwo

Babaláwo, another name for Yorùbá Traditional Healers of Nigeria, literally means "father of the secrets" (Epega & Neimark, 1995, p. xii). Mákindé (1974) posited that the *babaláwo* are undoubtedly men and women whose intelligence appears to be distinctly sharper than that of most of their followers.

They take keen delight in the recitation of their proverbs, songs, and wise sayings. Their influence is very extensive, as they are consulted in all the major affairs of life including social, psychological, physiological, intellectual, and political areas: "The *babaláwo* of the *Ifá* tradition predict events by focusing on individuals" (Epega & Neimark, 1995, p.vii). *Babaláwo*, like other effective helpers, know themselves and their clients very well. *Babaláwo* and Yorùbá Traditional Healers, consisting of both herbalists (*oníṣègùn*) and diviners (*Ifá* priests), are used synonymously in this study.

Divining

This is the traditional healers' method of predicting their clients' futures, by utilizing the divining chain to inquire concerning the future or the nature of their clients' problems from *Ifá (Ọ̀rúnmìlà)*. *Ọ̀rúnmìlà*, also referred to as *Ifá*, was one of the four hundred and one divinities who was sent by *Olódùmarè* (*the* Yoruba High God) from *Ọ̀run* (heaven) to *ayé* (earth) to assume certain responsibilities (Abímbọ̀lá, 1977). "It is through the vision and direction of *Ọ̀rúnmìlà's* words known as the sacred *odù*, that his wisdom and guidance are expressed on earth" (Epega & Neimark, 1995, p. xii). *Ọ̀rúnmìlà* (*Ifá*) was put in charge of divination because of his great wisdom which he acquired as a result of his presence by the side of *Olódùmarè*, when the latter created the universe (Abímbọ̀lá, 1977).

Epega & Neimark (1995) pointed out that "the training, knowledge, and spiritual insight of the practitioners are critical to the proper use of divination" (p.ix). These authors added that "a skilled *babaláwo* does not simply give a mechanical recitation of alternatives, [but] he carefully selects and blends the energy of the *odù* with the client's unique situation and works from there" (Epega & Neimark, 1995, p.ix). In the same vein, Abímbọ̀lá (1977) maintained that some clients consult *Ifá* at critical moments of their lives, including marriage, divorce, change of profession or place of abode.

Diviners

The *Yorùbá* refer to a diviner as one who predicts accurately (*aláfọ̀se*) and as one who predicts or tells before ṭhe problem emerges (*alásọtẹ́lẹ̀*). They are *Ifá* priests (*babaláwo*) who act as *Ọ̀rúnmìlà's* mouth piece among the *Yorùbá*. Diviners are the ones who utilize the *ọ̀pèlè* (divining chain) to inquire into and relay messages from *Ifá* to their clients. *Yorùbá* diviners consult *Ifá* and recite *Odù Ifá* as they unravel the problems of each of their clients "through specific ritual or offerings, which are indicated through divination" (Epega & Neimark, 1995, p. ix).

Babaláwo (*Ifá* priests) accomplish their goals through their ability to communicate and interpret the 256 *odù*, or sacred stories, of *Ifá* which have survived through thousands of years of oral tradition (Epega & Neimark, 1995). Epega & Neimark (1995) concluded that "in casting a specific *odù* for a client, the *babaláwo* (*Ifá* priest) meshes the universal energy and wisdom of the particular *odù* with the specific circumstances facing the client," and that "it is the "marriage" between the truth of the *odù* and the reality of the client that creates a unique and individual interpretation of current and future events" (p.ix).

Herbalists

These traditional healers utilize locally prepared herbs and concoctions to cure different diseases and ailments brought to them by clients. They are referred to as *adáhunṣe* or *oníṣègùn* in *Yorùbá* land and are respected for their innate and acquired knowledge, and ability to use different herbs to make medicaments for different diseases and illnesses (*wọ́n ní òye bí a ti í fi ewé ṣe oògùn).*

Traditional Counseling

Traditional counseling is seen by the *Yorùbá* people as a means by which traditional healers help them understand themselves and others, and ultimately enhance their personal satisfaction (Mallum, 1983). Traditional counseling is inherently embedded in *Yorùbá* tradition because people seek help for different problems from traditional healers as a way of living a holistic lifestyle and finding meaning for their lives.

Dean of Healers

These are the oldest and most respected *babaláwo* (*Ifá* priests and herbalists) who possess wide knowledge and experience of healing in *Yorùbá* land.

Odù Ifá

Odù Ifá comprises sixteen signs with 256 *odù*, chapters, or sacred stories of *Ifá* (Epega & Neimark, 1995, p. ix), parts of which are memorized by diviners (*Ifá* Priests). According to Epega & Neimark (1995), "the *odù* are powerful guides, with strong general characteristics, waiting to reach fruition as they apply to specific situations in our lives"(p. x).

Mákindé (1983) noted that these chapters (*odù*) comprise a vast compendium of knowledge, while Abímbọ̀lá (1968) referred to the *odù* as possessing the deepest wisdom and philosophy of the *Yorùbá* ethnic group. The sixteen primary *odù* are called *méjì*, or twos, with *Ejì Ogbè* as the first in the *Odù Ifá* series, while, *Ọ̀yèkú méjì* is the second in these series, with each *odù* carrying hundreds of tales that have accumulated in the oral tradition of *Ifá* (Epega & Neimark, 1995, p. xiii).

Ifá

The most dominant aspect of *Yorùbá* culture is associated with the oral and written *Ifá* literature. *Ifá* has challenging ideas that generate philosophical knowledge in metaphysics, ethics, epistemology, and science. *Ifá* knowledge progresses, is programmed and learned in 16 consecutive sets. The most complete and accurate form of *Ifá* divination can only be performed by a trained and initiated *Ifá* priest (Epega & Neimark, 1995).

Olu Mákindé (1983), a former dean of the Faculty of Education at Obáfémi Awólọ̀wò. University, a Nigerian counselor educator and an expert in the field of Yorùbá Traditional Healers, referred to *Ifá* as the repository of knowledge or the infinite source of knowledge (*ìmọ̀ àìmọ̀ tán*). Moreover, Akin Mákindé, the Head of the Philosophy Department at Ọbáfẹ́mi Awólówò. University in 1994, affirmed that *Ọ̀rúnmìlà (Ifá)* possesses knowledge of the following subjects: the study of nature (physics), animals (biology), plants (botany), oral incantations (*ọfọ̀*), divination (prediction), medicinal plants (herbalism), physiology (anatomy), and sciences associated with healing diseases (medicine)" (Mákindé, 1988). *Ifá* foretells by warning and provides solutions to anticipated events or problems. Mákindé (1984) observed that:

> Wisdom is known as *Ifá*
> knowledge is the other name for *Ọ̀pèlè Ifá*
> because we are bound to have problems.
> It is to be informed about something we are ignorant of
> that *Ifá* exists to help us (p. 88).

Divining Chain (*ọ̀pẹ̀lẹ̀*)

The divining chain (*ọ̀pèlè*) consists of "eight half seed shells held in the middle so that four shells fall in a line on each side" (Epega & Neimark, 1995, p.xv). Epega & Neimark (1995) added that "by casting the *ọ̀pèlè,* the *babaláwo* can, in a single toss, arrive at the necessary eight symbols to form a complete *odù*" (p.xv), thereby assisting clients to diagnose their problems and find appropriate solutions to these problems. However, they stated that the method of divining with the *ọ̀pèlè* is not as accurate or precise as divining with the *ikin.*

Alternative Medicine

Alternative medicine applies to various therapeutic systems not accepted by orthodox medical science because of their reported failure to submit to or withstand evaluation by objective methods such as the randomized clinical trial (Beeson & Scott, 1986). Techniques and disciplines that may be classified under alternative medicine include: homeopathy, osteopathy, chiropraxis, acupuncture, and herbal medicine (Beeson & Scott, 1986).

Moreover, Tratchman (1994) defined alternative medicine as being concerned with the qualities that distinguish people who may have the same diagnosis. Alternative medicine addresses the mental, emotional, and spiritual, as well as biological aspects of each person's life (Tratchman, 1994, p.116). Alternative medicine applies to various types of treatment used instead of established forms of modern medicine. Overall, it involves the continuous dissemination of healing methods of dynamic medical knowledge and ancestral experience.

Disease or Ill Health

Disease or ill health is induced by an imbalance or disequilibrium in a person's total ecological system (W.H.O., 1978). Disease occurs when someone is literally "without ease," and is defined as any sickness, ailment, or departure from the generally accepted norm of good health (Beeson & Scott, 1986). Overall, this study perceives disease or ill-health as being present when physical, psychological or emotional unease is apparent in a client's life.

Illness

Illness is present when an individual perceives herself or himself as diseased, and disease is present when identifiable by objective and external criteria.

Client

A client, for the purposes of this study, is a person who visits traditional healers, with psychological, physiological, organismic, or emotional problems, in the hope that his or her problem(s) will be solved.

Yorùbá

The *Yorùbá* are one of the largest ethnic groups in Africa. They are estimated to number 20.3 million, which is about 20 percent of Nigeria's population (Population Reference Bureau, 1995). They live predominantly in the southwestern part of Nigeria and have been divided by some geographers into over 20 subgroups including: *Ọyọ́, Ẹ̀gbá, Ikétu*, *Ọ̀họ̀rí, Ẹ̀gbádó, Ìjèbú, Ifè, Ìjèṣà*, *Ìgbóminà, Ondó,* and *Èkìtì* (Kurian, 1989, p. 283). *Yorùbá* settlements are characterized by their remarkable urban centers (Mábògùnjẹ, 1962), which are unparalleled anywhere else in tropical Africa.

Olódùmarè

The *Yorùbá* name for God Almighty, who created everything in the universe including the gods.

The gods

These are different categories of deities worshipped, prayed to and appeased by the *Yorùbá* people of Western Nigeria.

SUMMARY

The purpose of this research is to formulate hypotheses on how the interpersonal techniques used, as well as functions and roles performed, by Yorùbá Traditional Healers, impact the physical, interpersonal, interactional and inter-relational worlds of each of their clients and the total healing culture as a whole (Binswanger, 1962 & 1963). As a whole, this project utilized the case study approach to investigate the interpersonal techniques used by Yorùbá Traditional Healers.

Towards this end, this Chapter provided information on the formulation of hypotheses and a brief overview of the methodology utilized for the research project. Since the case study is mainly an inductive methodology, hypotheses are formulated, not tested. In Chapter Two of this volume, related literature on the Traditional healing systems and issues related to Yorùbá Traditional Healers and healing are reviewed. Chapter Three provides information on the methods and procedures that I utilized in conducting this study, while Chapters Four and Five discuss the profiled cases and hypotheses. Finally, Chapter Six summarizes my findings, and provides recommendations and related observations.

CHAPTER TWO

Review of Related Literature

THIS CHAPTER HIGHLIGHTS THE INTERACTIONAL AND INTERRELATIONAL roles and functions of, and the interpersonal techniques employed by, traditional healers. In this vein, the literature review presented herein specifically focuses on the following topics: Nigerian ethnic groups, *Yorùbá* land and the *Yorùbá*, ethno-medicine, personalistic and naturalistic etiologies, diagnoses in personalistic and naturalistic etiologies, disease and illness. Other reviewed concepts include alternative medicine, because it is a new approach of healing used in different parts of the world, cultural issues that are central to traditional healers' myths and superstitions, tradition, traditional systems of healing, helpers (traditional healers), roles and functions of traditional healers, herbalists and religious healers.

Themes such as traditional healers' techniques, props and cues, healing factors in traditional therapy, counseling and Western trained Nigerian counselors, as well as guidance and counseling in Nigeria, are all incorporated into the literature review and discussion. Quality and criticism of reviewed research are also discussed. The chapter ends with a summary of important points concerning the relevant roles and functions performed, and techniques used by traditional healers in all societies.

NIGERIAN ETHNIC GROUPS

Nigeria has a rich cultural heritage, deriving from its indigenous ethnic elements as well as from Middle Eastern and Western cultural influences. A typical African country in the diversity and heterogeneity of its ethnic heritage with more than 250 ethnic groups (Book of Facts, 1995), Nigeria is one of the most ethnically diverse countries in Africa and, relative to its size, in the world (World Almanac, 1995). The four dominant groups, *Igbo* in the East, *Yorùbá* in the West, and the *Hausa* and *Fulani* in the North constitute roughly 60 percent of the population. The *Igbo* have a population of approximately 16.6 million (17 percent), while the *Hausa* and *Fulani* have a population of 29.5 million (30 percent), and the *Yorùbá* have a population of 20.3 million (20 percent) (Population Reference Bureau, 1995).

Relative to Nigeria's population, the size of the non-African community, which is estimated at around 27,000, is small but diverse. The non-African community includes Britons, Americans, Lebanese, and Indians. Nigeria ranks seventh in the world in terms of ethnic and linguistic homogeneity, with 13 percent homogeneity (Europa, 1995).

YORÙBÁ LAND AND THE YORÙBÁ

Yorùbá land, located within the tropics, is closer to the equator than to the Tropic of Cancer. The roughly east-west coastline is on the average about 6 0' 22'N of the equator, where the coastline swings southwards towards the delta. The great achievement of *Yorùbá* settlements are their remarkable urban centers, unparalleled anywhere else in tropical Africa (Africa Yearbook, 1995), (Mábògùnjẹ́, 1962). *Yorùbá* indigenous economies revolve around hunting, fishing, farming, and craft industries, and members of the ethnic group have a long tradition of living in towns and cities (Population Reference Bureau, 1995), (Africa Yearbook, 1995), (Myers, 1989), (Òjó, 1967).

Epega & Neimark (1995) asserted that, "one of the great powers of the *Yorùbá* tradition is its ability to translate basic truth and wisdom through time, so that its application in our world of instant communication, high technology, and material goals and aspirations can be as accurate and beneficial today as it was thousands of years ago" (p.xvii). The *Yorùbá,* according to Mákindé (1974), have "their own distinct, systematic [sic] and rationalized ideas about the mysteries of the world; their philosophy is life affirming, be it true or mythical, scientific or not" (p.90).

He further reiterated that:

> the material endowment of the *Yorùbá* is a fund of invaluable information for the scientist. That the *Yorùbá* are so immeasurable above the apathy peculiar to the denizens of Western Africa in general, so vivacious and alert, so skillful in the management of life that they may very well be called the nation of practical philosophy of dusky African people who are ready with an apt illustration of whatever may be under discussion as the thoughtful peasant of Europe (p. 322).

The *Yorùbá,* Mákindé continued, are a people with their own philosophy of counseling with the *babaláwo* as the medium through which healing and counseling are practiced. *Babaláwo* are the traditional healers of *Yorùbá land,* comprising of diviners (*Ifá priests*) and herbalists (*Oníṣègùn* or *Adáhunṣe*).

ETHNOMEDICINE

Ethnomedicine is an area of study within the field of cultural anthropology that involves the comparative study of systems of medicine (Hughes, 1968). Ethnomedical systems are culturally unique beliefs and knowledge about health and disease held by the culture members, both health experts and nonexperts (McElroy & Townsend, 1985). Ethnomedicine analyzes society-wide as well as more localized, i.e., interpersonal, aspects of medical problems, with an emphasis on cultural factors (Fabrega, 1990).

An ethnomedical approach should illuminate how a society's culture creates and conditions specific problems involving health, illness, and medical practice. Levers & Maki (1994) contended that "the ethnomedical literature amplifies the importance of understanding the various paradigms of illness and health which are bound to culture, social construction, and, at least in part, to worldview" (p.12). Culturally-based beliefs about health and illness influence our interactions with people from other cultures, especially in health-care settings (Witte, 1991).

These subtle beliefs, which may be unknown to the health practitioner, might be obvious to the client. A person's socialization and cultural background form the framework from which he or she communicates. Feierman (1985) declared that the "evolution of health cannot be separated from the broader story of social change" (p.73). Additionally, "the political and economic forces which shaped the continent's [Africa] history also established the framework within which patterns of diagnosis and treatment, health and disease emerged" (Feierman, 1985, p.73).

Epega & Neimark (1995) maintained that the diviners' focus is on individual clients and the circumstances of their lives, not on their problems. These two authors added that shamans view the disease more as the problem, more than their clients or the circumstances of their clients' lives.

The biomedical perspective of Western medicine focuses more on the objective physiological processes of disease, while non-Western medical systems tend to focus more on the subjective perceptions of illness. Witte (1991) contended that no one medical system is right or correct, rather, each system provides a unique approach to understanding health and disease. Ethnomedicine has no developed theory of natural causation, while biomedicine treats social and psychological issues as secondary therapeutic problems (Morris, 1986).

Agyepong (1992) observed that ethnomedical perceptions of the causes of and treatment for malaria are different from conventional views among the *Adangbe* of Ghana. Many *Adangbe* perceived malaria as an environmentally-related disease caused by excessive contact with external heat which upsets the blood equilibrium. Therefore, many community members do not connect malaria with the mosquito, in theory or practice.

Personalistic and Naturalistic Etiologies

Personalistic and naturalistic etiologies are the two principal factors identified within the etiology of disease (Foster, 1976). Foster (1976) referred to disease etiology as the key to cross-cultural comparison in non-Western medical systems, and further explained that personalistic etiologies hold the belief that all misfortune, including disease, is explained in the same way: that illness, religion, and magic are inseparable. He stated that the most powerful healers have supernatural and magical powers, and that their primary role is diagnostic.

Scientific beliefs simply mingle with traditional ones instead of supplanting them (Roder, 1991). Beliefs in the supernatural causation of serious illness and death by sorcery, witchcraft, or taboo violation remain largely unchanged after Western medical methods were introduced in Papua New Guinea (Lepowsky, 1990). Foster (1976) explained that there is a belief that religion and magic are largely unrelated to illness, that the principal healers lack supernatural or magical powers, and that their primary role is therapeutic.

Most traditional healers in *Ilé-Ifẹ̀*, Nigeria, attributed deafness to supernatural causes, despite the distinction between congenital and non-congenital deafness (Ọdẹ́bíyì & Togonu-Bickersteth, 1987). Quidraogo (1989) also observed that traditional healers attributed illnesses to the will of God, witchcraft or magic.

Under the personalistic etiology, disease is explained as the results of the active purposeful intervention of an agent, who may be human (a witch or a sorcerer), nonhuman (a ghost, an ancestor, or an evil spirit), or supernatural (a deity or other very powerful being) (Foster, 1976). The sick person is literally a victim, the object of aggression or punishment directed specifically against him or her for reasons that concern him or her alone. Personalistic causality allows little room for accident or chance. If the agent intended harm to the victim, the etiology is commonly personalistic (Foster, 1976).

Illness is said to be but a special case in the explanation of all misfortunes in personalistic systems, while personalistic medical etiologies are parts of more comprehensive or general explanatory systems. Most authors agree, however, that clients, because of their beliefs in supernatural interventions, consult traditional healers for illnesses and diseases that have personalistic etiologies as their cause. Foster (1976) stated that most villagers believe that illness ultimately comes from God.

Naturalistic etiologies are, on the other hand, the belief that disease causality has nothing to do with other misfortunes. This naturalistic concept presupposes that religion and medical practices are almost inseparable. A possible reason for the persistence of these beliefs is that education and health services for Africans were for many years the exclusive province of Christian missions (Roder, 1991). Roder (1991) reiterated that western "civilization" was presented to Africans as a superior gift from a truer god, and not as a rational, logical, and scientific approach to life.

Illness is explained in impersonal systemic terms under naturalistic etiology. Disease is thought to stem not from the machinations of an angry being, but rather from such natural forces or conditions as cold, heat, winds, dampness, and above all, by a disruption in the balance of the basic body elements. The *yin,* the feminine passive principle in nature exhibited in Chinese cosmology in darkness, cold or wetness, combines with *yang,* the masculine active principle exhibited in light, heat or dryness, to produce an equilibrium. Health conforms to and results in an equilibrium model, when the humors, the *yin* and *yang* or the *Ayurvedic dosha,* are in the balance appropriate to the age and condition of the individual in his natural and social environment (Foster, 1976). Clients consult traditional healers and Western-trained medical doctors for diseases and illnesses that are explained within the realm of naturalistic etiologies.

DIAGNOSIS IN PERSONALISTIC ETIOLOGIES

Personalistic systems see the shaman or witch doctor diagnoses in terms of trance or other divinatory techniques. Diagnosis—to find out who and why—is the primary skill that the patient seeks from the curer. Treatment of the instrumental cause, while important, is of secondary concern (Foster, 1976).

The basic personal health strategy in personalistic etiologies emphasizes the importance of ensuring that one's social networks with fellow human beings, with ancestors, and deities are maintained in good working order. Time and money are essential ingredients in the maintenance of health in personalistic etiologies. Clients invest in money and time for rituals to God, ancestors and the gods.

DIAGNOSIS IN NATURALISTIC ETIOLOGIES

Naturalistic systems view diagnosis as being of very minor importance, as far as the curer is concerned. Diagnosis is made, not by the curer, but by the client and the members of his or her family. For instance, the initial psychiatric interview is usually a group activity where all significant members, friends, and co-workers present are invited to participate (Asuni, 1990). Treatment is based on findings of physical and mental state examinations, and focused on drawing relatives' attention to unhealthy interactions (Asuni, 1991). Asuni further reiterated that the discharge procedure and follow-up are also addressed and the client returns to the time prior to when the illness was diagnosed. For example, Foster (1976) recalled how the fact that he stepped on a cold wet floor the night before caused "risen heat" (p. 780).

Moreover, as pointed out earlier, the *Adangbe* of Ghana believe that malaria is an environmentally-related disease caused by excessive contact with external heat which upsets the blood equilibrium (Agpeyong, 1992), instead of by the mosquito as proved by modern Western medicine. In Guyarat, India, diarrhea is attributed to the excessive consumption of hot foods (Pool, 1987).

Overall, Foster (1976) felt that naturalistic etiologies correlate predominantly with "don'ts," which means that in theory, a hypercautious individual should be able to avoid almost all illnesses by "not doing certain things" (p.780). In contrast, personalistic systems emphasize the "dos." The naturalistic system emphasizes knowledge of how the system works and the will to live according to its dictates (Foster, 1976).

DISEASE

Disease is an objective phenomenon of organic malfunction, e.g., bacterial infection, viral attack, or injury (Witte, 1991). However, Rankin (1993) argued that individuals of various cultures have different perspectives about sickness and health. Foster (1976) declared that the culture in which people are socialized determines the beliefs that they hold concerning the nature of their problems and the way they may be solved.

McKee (1987) propounded two theories of causality. One theory of disease causality seeks explanations of pathogenesis in supernatural interventions or humorous imbalances; the other theory rests firmly on the germ theory of disease. The primary approaches to health and disease can be explained within sociological perspectives. The structural concept reveals disease as being dysfunctional, because it threatens the equilibrium by affecting normative and valued social participation in societal activities (Alonzo, 1984). An ideational/interactional perspective focuses specifically on the process of disease definition and evaluation and on their social consequences (Alonzo, 1984).

Supposedly, disease results from the normally and naturally-emergent changes in the environment and our inability to meet these ever-emerging changes in our socially-produced environment (Alonzo, 1984). The image of health, expressed by Dubos (1959), is that of a relationship to one's social, psychological, and physical environments. Diviners seek the underlying etiology of disease or misfortune among their African clients through reference to social conflicts or moral transgressions (Morris, 1986).

Epidemics are popularly explained in many villages as being the result of the wrath of a malevolent goddess (such as *Sitala* in India) associated with smallpox, measles, and other febrile diseases characterized by skin eruptions (Weiss, 1986). Evil spirits or familiar spirits have both been purported to be the cause of disease in 'traditional' societies. Traditional healers are believed to be the only agents who can remove these spirits from their victims (Green, 1985). It is because of this trust in traditional healing that sexually transmitted diseases in Africa are always presented to traditional healers, because clients and healers seem to believe that cures effected by the latter are more effective than modern cures (Green, 1992).

Illness

Illness is an individual's perception of not feeling well. Someone can have a disease yet not feel ill, e.g., hypertension. On the other hand, one can feel ill but not have a disease, e.g., psychosomatic illnesses. Usually, however, one experiences disease and illness simultaneously, e.g., the flu, cancer, or infection.

Illness is a recurring phenomenon in human groups and social factors, as opposed to molecular variables alone, must be considered when analyzing its causes (Dossey, 1994). Non-Western and small-scale societies tend to conceptualize illness holistically with wide ranging meanings. Two classes of religious explanations for mental illness among the *Annang* of Nigeria, possession and non-possession, were identified in the sociocultural milieu of the people (Umoren, 1990).

According to Fabrega (1990), illness brings fundamental concerns of a people, such as community rivalries, antagonisms, and relations with spiritual agencies, "to the fore." Treatment is often a highly-socialized spectacle with potentially-religious, moral, and political impacts on clients. Although the *Igbo* of Nigeria use both kinds of health care services in tandem, modern medicine is generally regarded as a secondary approach (Ezeji & Sarvela 1992). These authors added that there is a general feeling that illness management is never complete until a traditional management is undertaken.

Distinctions between mental and bodily illnesses are not generally produced (Ezeji & Sarvela). In some more complex and small-scale societies, one finds genuine specialists dealing with mental illness. Generally, however, non-specialist practitioners treat different types of illness, including those classified as psychiatric and psychological. Fabrega (1990) affirmed that the theory of illness of the early modern era was also eclectic. Problems that were labeled as psychopathological were handled in social-psychological and religious terms, with the family and community as active agents in their management and treatment.

Notions of illness causation are an important issue in the comparative study of medical systems. A review of literature on this topic reveals that etiological knowledge in non-Western cultures is dominated by religious or supernatural beliefs, in contrast to the supposedly more scientific and rational "Western etiological system" (Ngokwey, 1988, p. 793). However, there are exceptions even in the West. Waldram (1990) found that native residents of a western Canadian city retain a strong belief in traditional illness etiologies and the efficacy of traditional medicine. These western Canadian residents refer to creator, witchcraft, and ancestor spirits as the causes of illness.

Illness in Swaziland is believed to be sorcery-induced and environmentally-caused, i.e., diseases are thought to be in the air or in its agents. Illness could be caused by magical poisons that are hidden by one's enemies in places that a victim is likely to walk past or touch (Green, 1985). Beliefs about supernatural or mystical causation of mental illness and the efficacy of modern psychiatric resources versus traditional healers are also prevalent in Turkey (Eskin, 1989).

Nigerians and other Africans also believe that illness is caused by the deliberate use of spells and harmful medicines or, less commonly, by ancestral displeasure resulting in the withdrawal of spiritual protection (Green, 1985). Certain *Yorùbá* healers interviewed in Ọdejídé, Ọlátawúrà, Sàndà and Oyènẹ́yẹ́'s (1978) study characterized curse (*Èpè*) (75.5 percent), mysterious epidemic infections *(Ṣànpọ̀nná)* (67.9 percent), spirits (*Ànjọ̀nú*) (47.2 percent), and heredity (*Ìran*) (32.2 percent), as the etiological causes of mental illness in the city of *Ìbàdàn*, Ọ̀yọ́ State. Eight of the 53 *Yorùbá* healers interviewed stressed the importance of conflicts of the mind as a possible etiological factor. Overall, traditional healers attributed illnesses to the will of God or to witchcraft (Quidraogo, 1989).

For their part, the *Pokot* of Kenya perceive illness causation as a dynamic phenomenon embracing various planes of reality. They believe that it is possible for the same illness to be caused by natural physio-chemical processes, social, and spiritual forces. The client's pathological condition provides the starting point for the process of illness causation (Nyamwaya, 1987), which may be divided into the "how" and the "why" dimensions (Pritchard, 1937). The "how" dimension alludes to natural, physio-chemical, and psychological causes such as old age, bad air, moisture, thunder, and organisms, while the "why" plane regards social and spiritual relationships as directing or aggravating an illness.

Nyamwaya (1987) concluded that it has become increasingly clear that concepts of causality are crucial in determining the relationship between traditional and modern Western-based medicine, particularly in the initial stages of contact. Concepts and causality become less important in influencing the relationship at the latter stages of contact. Some illnesses purportedly are uniquely African and therefore not treatable by Western medicine (Nyamwaya, 1987). Similarly, Rankin & Kappy (1993) argued that health care professionals must be aware that individuals of different cultures may have perspectives about sickness and health that differ from theirs.

Certain African-Americans, Hispanic-Americans, and Native-Americans use unconventional therapies or traditional treatments (Rankin & Kappy, 1993). Furthermore, Ecuadorians believe that "evil eye," "evil air," and "soul loss," which are all classified as supernatural attacks, are illnesses not treatable by Western doctors (McKee, 1987). Ecuadorians believe that the above diseases must be treated by different methods deemed appropriate by traditional medicine.

Healing is required for a wide range of problems that includes not only physical ailments for middle-class suburban Americans, but their emotional, spiritual, and social dimensions as well (Kantor, 1993). Kantor's study of healing narratives broadened the discussion of health and illness, and supported previous research undertaken in other countries. She further noted that, for middle-class Americans, illness is not just an unpleasant reality of life, it necessitates an explanation and resolution, and is something to be overcome and conquered.

Comaroff (1980) defined healing as "fundamentally concerned with the reconstitution of physical, social, and spiritual order... [and that] ... it cannot be meaningfully examined if isolated from the wider sociocultural system" (p. 639). Additionally, Levers & Maki (1994) stated that anthropological literature informs us about how Africans become ill and seek healing rather than treatment. Hence, social factors must be considered to understand health and illness (Dossey, 1994), since religious and political beliefs, as well as attitudes toward alternative medicine, were the most consistent and powerful predictors of health-related beliefs (Furnham, 1994).

Alternative Medicine

The tendency to focus on the whole person has been postulated to be the reason why clients seek healers or experts for alternative healing methods (Cassidy, 1994; Murray and Shepherd 1993; Trachtman, 1994). Specialists in modern medicine, according to Trachtman (1994), have a limited view of the world, while generalists, who have an alternative view of medicine or healing, see more of the whole person. Generally, alternative medicine is concerned with the qualities that distinguish people who may have the same diagnosis, and it addresses the mental, emotional, spiritual, and biological aspects of each person's life (Trachtman, 1994). In highlighting the credibility of alternative medicine, Gellert (1994) posited that alternative healers tend to suggest that they are "cure-alls."

Murray & Shepherd (1993) claimed that women express more interest than men in alternative healing practices. After having interviewed males and females for their study, they found that the use of non-conventional care was associated with higher general practice consultation rates among women. Other variables, including age, religion, political beliefs, and beliefs regarding health and illness, also influence clients' preferences for alternative methods of healing (Furnham, 1994).

Those who consult alternative practitioners typically believed that their treatment should concentrate on the whole person and that their practitioners had greater knowledge of the physiology of the body (Furnham & Forey's (1994). Individuals interviewed for Furnham and Forey's study were more critical and skeptical about the efficacy of modern medicine, believed their health could be improved, stayed loyal to their chosen practitioner, tried more alternative therapies, and had more ecologically-aware lifestyles.

Cultural Issues

Culture

Hoebel (1972) defined culture as "the integrated system of learned behavior patterns characteristic of the members of a society which are not the result of biological inheritance" (p.6), while Tylor (1989) viewed culture as that complex whole which includes knowledge, belief, art, law, custom, other capabilities, and habits acquired by man as a member of society. Who we are and what we do is determined by our biological heritage, our natural surroundings, the group in which we live, and the means, the knowledge, the skills, and the ways of behaving, by which the members of our group function together to satisfy mutual requirements (Cone & Pelto, 1969).

The culture in which people are socialized determines the beliefs that they hold about the nature of their problems and how they may be solved (Vontress, 1991). Vontress conceded that African clients' beliefs affect the extent to which they consider the counselor's intervention strategies beneficial. This last point is particularly helpful when considering why African clients consult traditional healers.

Medicine and therapy are more clearly a function of the culture than of environmental conditions (Lámbò, 1983; Ackerkrecht, 1943). This is one of the reasons why Rankin and Kappy (1993) advocated a program that fosters cross-cultural education for individuals of different cultures, by enhancing cultural awareness and recognizing traditional healers' roles through lectures, workshops, and resident rotations.

Cultural misunderstandings and conflicts occur when two persons with differing cultural orientations assume that they share the same expectations for a situation but employ different behaviors to convey their intentions (Pedersen and Pedersen, 1989). This is an important variable to consider during cross-cultural interactions between clients and counselors.

Cultural variables can intervene in a counseling interview in at least three different ways (Pedersen, 1983): one is through the culture of the client; another is through the culture of the counselor; and a third is through the culture of the "problem." The problem defines the context of a counseling interview and assumes characteristics from the cultural context. A problem is a very complex configuration that draws from the total environment of the client, persons significant to the client, and perhaps even from the counselor who becomes much like an artificial personality to the client. Finally, a problem is perceived as an "independent" force with an independent identity (Pedersen, 1983).

A triadic or three-pronged relationship exists between the counselor, client, and an invisible but ever-present third party—culture (Saleh, 1986). Culture is a fluid factor, not a stagnant one, and varies according to the specific counseling relationship (Saleh, 1989), which is the spatial distance in cultural congruence between a counselor and his or her client.

Culture enters the relationship through the counselor and the 'counselee' since both are culturally imbued. The counselor utilizes tools such as training, methods, techniques, theories, and approaches in the counseling relationship. Culture acts as an agent that either predisposes the relationship to a successful outcome or contributes to the dooming of the relationship. Culture has made a profound contribution to our understanding of human behavior through explanations of personal development and interpersonal contact (Pedersen & Pedersen, 1989). Rather than refer to a person's culture as an external factor in a counseling relationship, an accurate assessment must relate culture to the client's intended expectations and values (Pedersen & Pedersen, 1989).

Since no one is culture-free, and it is highly unlikely that any one cultural viewpoint will fit everyone's needs, there is a need to include cultural aspects of counseling into all counselor education programs (Saleh, 1989). As each culture is distinct, counseling must acknowledge and respond in a nurturing manner to the cultural differences existing within the world's population before its applicability can be carried beyond its self-imposed, mono-cultural encasement (Boas, 1964).

Studies in psychology, linguistics, and anthropology all point to the same conclusion: people think differently (Torrey, 1986). Torrey stressed that all men apparently do not see things in the same way, and that culture determines the way they see things. Differences in perception are superficial and include such basic things as colors and numbers. In sum, cultural notions imply differences in thought at all levels including ideas, values, conceptions of time, and the notion of cause and effect (Torrey, 1986).

Culture and Traditional Healers

Ìdòwù (1985) stipulated that for any healing system to be meaningful and effective for Africans it must give prominence to their cultural background. African healers focus on stimulating their clients' healing powers by associating their belief systems with their emotional and body states (Ìdòwú, 1985). Efforts are being made in Rwanda (and other parts of the world) to integrate traditional medicine with modern methods (Baro, 1990). Integrating western medical practice with indigenous health care is also advocated as a viable source of holistic health for the *Igbo* of Nigeria (Ezeji & Sarvela, 1992).

Myths and Superstitions

One Zimbabwean traditional healer interviewed by Levers & Maki (1994) asserted, "myths serve a function in society" (p.63). According to Ìdòwú (1985), such myths and superstitions are transmitted from one generation to another through the process of acculturation. They are both expressed and reinforced through recurring group activities, e.g., dances, religious ceremonies, and rituals. African myths and superstitions provide living symbols of the history, the culture, and the daily practices of Africans. They also portray the hopes and fears of Africa's people as they struggle to understand the unknown and to combat the stresses of their environment.

Ìdòwú (1985) found that African theories are created and beliefs are constructed through myths and superstition, which form the cornerstone of traditional African healing. Myths are developed in Africa to explain:

(a) Human phenomena, e.g., creation, death, illness, disease, and relationships among people (including the dead);
(b) Natural occurrences, e.g., rain; or
(c) Disasters, e.g., famine, drought, and epidemics (Ìdòwú, 1985, p. 83).

African myths and superstitions also serve other purposes. They foster socialization and help to counteract anxiety caused by ontological beliefs or by the prospect of disappearing into nothingness (Frank, 1978). Myth and superstition further engender psychological, emotional, and mental well-being (Ìdòwú, 1985), but the effects on emotional states can only be inferred and not scientifically validated. Frank (1978) noted that:

> in order to select among and make sense out of the welter of experiences, humans need a moral and cognitive map of the universe. Such maps may be termed belief systems (or myths) and they include beliefs as to the nature of knowledge and code of ethics—that is—descriptions of valued and devalued behaviors. Ultimately, all belief systems rest on premises which are not open to question and which cannot be demonstrated empirically—that is, they are articles of faith (p. 260).

Ìdòwú (1985) hinted that myths and superstitions act as forces of cultural integration and awareness, and promote community cohesiveness. He confirmed that elders educate people, especially youth, about the culture and its ancestry. Myths and superstitions entertain and work as a cathartic component, act as mythological tales, and are used as songs to evoke emotions and reduce anxiety.

As previously noted, deafness is attributed to superstitions among 98 Yorùbá Traditional Healers interviewed in *Ilé-Ifẹ̀*, Nigeria (Ọdẹ́bíyì & Togonu-Bickersteth, 1987). Myths and superstitions allay the fears of clients from the healers' perspective, and situate clients' problems in proper cultural perspectives. Ọdẹ́bíyì (1989) remarked that healers also use food taboos to explain children' problems to their mothers as a way of assuaging their fears.

TRADITION

Tradition is a belief or practice in any field of culture, to the extent that it is received from the hands, lips, or examples of others rather than being discovered or invented. The assumption is that the authors and transmitters are reliable, and, therefore, the tradition is valid.

Eliade (1987) divided tradition into verbal and nonverbal. Verbal tradition includes traditional artifacts (e.g., icons, monuments, and symbolic objects), sites, designs, gestures, postures, customs, and institutions. Nonverbal traditions, on the other hand, cannot exist in isolation from verbal traditions, because the latter are needed for interpretation. Tradition, like traditional healing, is an indirect source of knowledge that is not readily accessible to or verifiable from contemporary sources.

TRADITIONAL SYSTEMS OF HEALING

Traditional systems of medicine contribute significantly to the medical needs of 80 per cent of the world's population (WHO, Technical Reports 622, 1978). The WHO (1976) defined traditional medicine as the comprehensive "knowledge and practices, whether explicable or not, used in diagnosis, prevention and elimination of physical, mental or social disequilibrium and relying exclusively on practical experience and observation handed down from generation to generation, verbally or in writing" (p.3).

Traditional methods of healing have been employed by a majority of the world's population for thousands of years (Tratchman, 1994). African traditional medicine existed before the introduction of Western medicine, and suited the needs of African cultures (Mákindé, 1988). Tratchman (1994) contended further that ignoring the contributions of traditional healers is tantamount to technological arrogance. Theories and practices of medicine have a clear cultural dimension, as the traditional systems and policy emerged from the beliefs and cultures of Africans (Mákindé, 1988). According to Mákindé (1988), this occurred because the majority has faith in the power and efficacy of traditional medicine. Patients seem to believe that traditional cures are more effective than modern cures (Green, 1992). Levers & Maki (1994) discovered that in Swaziland "with traditional beliefs and practices, even when people go to the hospital, they would rather go and see a traditional healer" (p.52).

The efficacy of Western medicine is not disputed in Africa or Asia (including India or China) but the traditional system is also highly in demand (Mákindé, 1988). In Nigeria, millions of patients in both urban and rural areas depend on traditional healing for treatment (Mákindé, 1988). The majority of Africans in rural areas look for treatment of diseases and illness (including mental illness) from traditional healers who share their experience and culture and thereby understand their problems. Consequently, the first point of contact for health concerns for most Africans is the traditional healer; they spend more time with healers than with Western doctors (Levers & Maki, 1994; Dillon-Malone, 1988; Feierman, 1985; Gay, 1993; Gay & Gill, 1993; Janzen, 1992; & Vontress, 1991).

HELPERS

Traditional Healers

Traditional healing is as old as the human race. Indigenous healers were prevalent amongst the Egyptians, early humans, and in the old civilizations of Greece and the Roman Empire (Schusky & Culbert, 1967). The former Director of WHO in Lesotho claimed, "there are over one million traditional healers in southern Africa, with about ½ million of those practicing in the Republic of South Africa" (Levers & Maki, 1994, p. 46).

Traditional healers are successful with their clients because they share the same worldview, possess the ability to diagnose problems, have distinct personality characteristics, and have a reputation that helps raise their clients' expectations (Torrey, 1986). Torrey added that traditional healers utilize techniques that generate emotional arousal and give these clients a sense of mastery over their problems.

Indigenous healers are equipped to provide health care within different communities (WHO, 1978). These healers may use vegetable, animal, and mineral substances in their healing practices, and their methods may be "based on the social, cultural and religious backgrounds, as well as the knowledge, attitudes and beliefs that are prevalent in the community regarding physical, mental and social well being and the causation of disease and disability" (WHO, 1978, p.41).

Traditional healers are held in high regard because of their ability to exploit the forces of nature and make contact with the spirit world (Vontress, 1991). Healers vary in terms of their power to heal. They are generally viewed as holistic, because of their ability to serve as a priest-physician-psychologist (Vontress, 1991). They perform religious functions of healing and therapeutic duties concurrently, when there is need for it.

Africans have faith in diviners, other traditional healers and herbalists, as well as in medicinal plants (Ṣófowórà, 1981). In a special message to the now-defunct Organization of African Unity (O. A. U.) meeting in Lagos, Nigeria, Abdel Razik, its erstwhile Assistant Executive Secretary, affirmed that Africans prefer traditional medicine to modern medicine and western-based counseling methods (Ṣófowórà, 1981).

Nigerians consult western trained doctors for their health problems and also seek out traditional healers who deal with the metaphysical issues that supposedly underlie physical complaints (Roder, 1991). In Lesotho, people come to healers when "things are not going well ... and when they are physically sick" (Levers & Maki, 1994, p.44). Africans generally consult specialists such as the herbalist, the fetish man, the medium, the healer, and the sorcerer (Vontress, 1991). Two broad categories of indigenous traditional health practitioners include those who are possessed (by supernatural powers or the spirit of the ancestral healer), including the spiritual healer, the fortune teller, and the clairvoyant, and those who are non-possessed, including the traditional doctors, the medicine men and the herbalists (Levers & Maki, 1994). Vontress (1991) also posited that African specialists differ in terms of knowledge, magical powers, and focus.

The herbalist is an individual who knows the medicinal qualities of herbs (Vontress, 1991), while the fetish man is one who manipulates great powers. The mediums are individuals, mostly women, who are usually endowed with the power to transmit messages from the dead to the living (Stoller, 1989). Healers are considered by Mbiti (1988) to be generalists referred to in Francophone Africa as "*le guerisseur*." Anglophone countries (of which Nigeria is one), simply refer to healers as "medicine men," "*jùjú* men," "traditional healers," "witch doctors" or "*babaláwo*" (Mbiti, 1988).

Awanbor (1982) explains that the *Edo* people of Nigeria use the general term *obos* to refer to native doctors, similar to the term *babaláwo* among the *Yorùbá*. Mákindé (1984), identified the following group of indigenous counseling practitioners: "*uzenakpo* (those who help people out of problems) among the *Ibiobio*; *dibia*, *bokaye*, and *ogbafa* among the *Igbo*; *omufunmu* among the *Bugisu* of Uganda; *nganga* in Tanzania; *sikidy* in Malagasy; *obozi* among the Igala-Tiv; and *babaláwo* among the *Yorùbá*" (p. 87). These traditional healers are regarded as "poets Lucretius of ancient wisdom" within their respective communities (Mákindé, 1984, p. 87).

Traditional practitioners provide health care for an average of 75 percent of the population in the developing world, including Nigeria (Ṣófowórà, 1981). This underscores the necessity of considering this class of health practitioners. Ṣófowórà (1981) stated that international organizations like the World Health Organization (WHO), United Nation Industrial Development Organization (UNIDO), United Nations Children's Emergency Fund (UNICEF), Economic Community of West African States (ECOWAS) and the African Union (AU) now have major programs for the development of traditional medicine in Africa. These efforts help to enhance holistic health for people in different parts of the world.

There is approximately one traditional *nganga* for every 350 residents of Dar es Salaam, the capital of Tanzania; the number is probably higher in rural areas (Rappaport, 1977). Since 80 percent of the Nigerian rural population lack access to Western-trained doctors, nurses, midwives, and other paramedical health workers (Oyèbọlá, 1980), traditional healers are the major available source of health care.

Traditional counselors are not just people who advise but men and women who offer activities, have fame or prestige, and proffer cultural or mythical explanations that are inherently psychological in nature (Mallum, 1983). Traditional healers are associated with religion, spirits, supernatural powers and the gods; people refer to such individuals as native doctor or divinator, medicine-man, witch-doctor, herbalist, soothsayer or seer (Mallum, 1983). They are also called sorcerer, magician or occultist, depending on the functions that they perform. Mallum (1983) also stated that it is this traditional healer or native doctor, as educated Nigerians refer to them, that the people choose as their traditional counselor when they experience problems.

Clients with problems ranging from maladjustment to infertility visit traditional healers for counseling, diagnosis, discovery of etiology, or the pathogenic agent at work, as well as initiating catharsis, finding solutions and predicting their future and fortunes. These traditional healers also take care of other problems, like revealing the past, finding lost articles, engendering self-actualization, and progress in endeavors (Mallum, 1983). The top 10 diseases treated by traditional healers in Swaziland were as follows: wounds, Sexually Transmitted Diseases (STDs), kidney and bladder problems, virility for men, stomach complaints, high blood pressure, diarrhea, female complaints and colic (Levers & Maki, 1994). A female traditional healer in Swaziland reportedly treated hematological diseases, psychiatric disorders, dental problems, and sometimes polio as well (Levers & Maki, 1994).

In order to improve the health of all Malawians, MacLachlan (1993) advocated increased collaboration between traditional healers and western trained mental health practitioners. Traditional healers can be utilized in community-based AIDS education since they hold roles of authority in the social networks in poor urban communities (Schoepf, 1992; Hickson & Mokhobo, 1992). The authors reiterated that traditional healers' pragmatism may be more effective to Malawians than the moralistic teachings of intellectuals.

Asuni (1990) was also of the opinion that the use of traditional healers to prevent, educate and treat mental illness as a family and group affair will go a long way to foster holistic health among Nigerians. Ọdẹ́jídè, Ohaeri, Adélẹkàn and Ikuesan (1989) agreed that traditional healers can foster growth among clients in the treatment and prevention of and education on, alcoholism in Nigeria.

Abas, Broadhead, Mmbape and Khumalo-Sakatukwa (1994) discussed the critical role that traditional healers assume in the treatment of depression in Zimbabwe, while Ezeji & Sarvela (1992) observed that modern medicine is generally regarded as a secondary approach to traditional methods among the *Igbo* of Nigeria. Consequently, traditional healing methods, modern counseling methods, and medicine could be integrated for the general benefit of mankind because they are complementary (Baro, 1990; N'donazi, 1991; & Quidraogo, 1989; Mákindé, 1988). Modern pharmacists also have a lot to gain from traditional healers by understudying their herbal knowledge (N'donazi, 1991).

Babaláwo (generic name for Yorùbá Traditional Healers) attend promptly to clients' needs (Mákindé, 1974). As demonstrated in Chapters Four and Five, their work involves information giving, educational and vocational planning, as well as preventive, rehabilitative and developmental tasks. Mákindé (1973) stated that their training is long and inclusive: "Realizing their balanced training, high motivation, acceptance in the community, and willingness to help solve problems, there is no doubt that their methods and philosophies should be borrowed for individual counseling in West Africa" (p. 326).

In recognition of the innate utility of alternative therapies, the National Institutes of Health (NIH) has evaluated lifestyle programs like macrobiotics, vegetarian, natural foods diet, food supplements, and such well known approaches to managing stress as yoga, and breathing and relaxation techniques, prayer, biofeedback, visualization, art or music therapies and acupuncture from China (Trachtman, 1994). Indigenous practices from other cultures, like *Ayur Veda* from India, homeopathy, native American practices and microdose pharmacology from Europe, are among the traditional healing practices that have been researched at the NIH.

Roles and Functions of Traditional Healers

Western and traditional healing systems have come into greater contact with each other since the WHO pledged in 1977 that there should be provision of worldwide health care by the year 2000 (Krippner, 1984). This was to become practical through the training of native healers, and their incorporation into Western medical clinics and hospitals. It was also recommended that Malawian students obtain training in traditional mental health services for students in Malawi as part of their medical education (MacLachlan, 1993).

Healers are depicted by Vontress (1991) as consultants for physical and psychological problems. N'donazi (1991) revalidated the healing wisdom of traditional healers in his study of the *Souma* healers of Central Africa. Diallo and Hall (1989) also claimed that people from the *Igbo* and *Yorùbá* ethnic groups of Nigeria often perceive physical and mental illness as resulting from contact with evil spirits who may have been provoked by the violation of the visible or invisible order.

The healer acts in part as an intermediary between these visible and invisible worlds to determine which spirits are at work and how to bring the ill client back into harmony with them (Vontress, 1991). Veyrat and Ferrier (1989) contended that ritual-dominated traditional healing is the most appropriate and effective treatment regimen for psychosomatic patients from magic-dominated cultures. While Western education and modern medicine have made great headway in Africa, beliefs in witchcraft and traditional medicine flourish alongside the newer ideas (Roder, 1991). As such clients still consult traditional healers who deal with metaphysical issues (Roder, 1991).

Abas et al. (1994) averred that traditional healers play a key role in helping clients defeat depression in Zimbabwe. Traditional healers also assist in community-based AIDS education in Zaire because they hold roles of authority in the country's social networks (Schoepf, 1992). Hickson & Mokhobo (1992) supported the above point by stating that traditional healers' skills should be used for effective AIDS prevention and cure. Levers & Maki (1994) further stated that healers in Zimbabwe use counseling for HIV/AIDS clients, "because it can enable the patient to cope with the current situation and to discuss whatever depression he or she is experiencing as a result" (p.64). Traditional healers also assist and heal by reconstructing a patient's personality in a renewed harmonious relationship within the social support network (Auge, 1989).

Dr. Thomas A. Lámbò (1983), a renowned Nigerian and Western-trained psychiatrist, declared that in talking of African medicine:

> the concepts of health and disease can be regarded as constituting a continuous transition with almost imperceptible gradations. In these and related cultures, the determinants of health and disease are conceptualized holistically. Psychotherapy… is an indispensable phase of a variety of institutionalized processes to promote human well-being. Because the healer plays a variety of roles in the community, he or she is able to address many different aspects of the problems of living brought by the client (p. 2).

He also made the following observation:

> Your rural witch doctor is, in addition to medicine man, something of a social and probation worker, teacher, priest, and JP (justice of the peace). He may tackle the problem, of which his patient's symptoms are only a part, with an across-the-board-approach impossible to the fragmented social, penal, and medical services in the West (Lámbò, 1974, pp. 33–34).

Levers & Maki (1994) added that "traditional practitioners have a holistic approach to the medicine they practice" (p. 63), and "traditional healing considers patients in holistic relationship to their environments" (p.74).

Herbalists' Role

Healers are acclaimed to have wide knowledge in the use of herbs (Krippner, 1984). In fact, the former WHO director recognized that "modern medicine has a great deal still to learn from the collector of herbs" (Krippner, 1984, p. 157). Healers' use of plants to cure many ailments, diseases and illness has been advantageous to western culture, which derives many medicines from African plants and herbs (N'donazi, 1991). Lepowsky (1990) opined that most islanders first utilize prepared herbs and plants from traditional healers before visiting western trained doctors and nurses' aides.

Root Bernstein, a physiologist and historian of ancient medical practices at Michigan State University, cited one example that can be verified by modern science: the treatment of injuries with sugar and honey, which are now known to prevent infection (McAuliffe, 1992). Thus, McAuliffe urged chemists in the pharmaceutical industry to study lesser-known herbs and other compounds whose curative properties have been extolled by witch doctors, shamans, and other traditional healers, so that modern medical experts can utilize them for the good of all.

Religious Healers

One of the most positive results of religious healing, according to Edwards (1983), is the creative reintegration of healing and religion. The *Yorùbá* believe in a spiritual being (referred to as *Olódùmarè*) higher than other forces. Religious healing practices exist side by side with traditional healing in Nigeria.

Religio-psychotherapeutic (including relaxation, suggestion and manipulation) and religio-physiologic practices (including the use of chains and tranquilizing medicine) are the two treatment modalities that Umoren (1990) enumerated as common with some syncretic religious healers in Nigeria. Ọdẹ́jídé, Ohaeri, Adélékàn and Ikuesan (1989) added that alcoholism is commonly treated with some recognized approaches in some Nigerian syncretic churches. Nigerians also consult religious healers and hold persistent beliefs in their capability to ensure good luck in farming, fishing, love, business and other pursuits because education and health services were for many years the exclusive province of Christian missions (Roder, 1991).

The Christian concept of healing sees God as a willful power who intervenes in this world to produce change in the sick person, and the healing ministry has much to do with the healing of the memory as the healing of the body (Easthope, 1986). The Christian faith may be understood to open the way to a greater sense of the potential for wholeness in the midst of disharmony and threat, through the experience of forgiveness and renewal in Christ and of living by the power of the Holy Spirit (Easthope, 1986).

The four areas that religious healers emphasize during healing are the physical, mental, emotional, and spiritual. The healer then lays hands on the client and feels in his or her own body exactly what is troubling the client to the point where the symptoms are actually transferred to the healer (Edwards, 1983). The religious healer gets an insight into what happens through prayer for enlightenment concerning the client's symptoms (diagnosis). Here, the healer experiences harmony with God, who is believed to be the source of knowledge and healing, and becomes deeply conversant with the client's needs.

The ability to diagnose different diseases allows religious healers to compare favorably with traditional healing methods. During a divination session, the indigenous healer demonstrates her or his ability to know the client's illness, without being told the symptoms, and his reputation rests in part at least on competence at doing this. The Holy Spirit is the source of religious healers' knowledge, while the traditional healers claim to divine the nature and cause of the affliction by communicating with ancestors and by consulting the *Ifá* oracle.

The first part of the religious healing session consists of worship, prayer, singing, confessions, and testimonies. The second part is Holy Bible reading and preaching, which leads to the third part where the clients present themselves for healing (Edwards, 1983). The religious healer emphasizes wholeness and the counseling function as an important part of healing. Healers do this through an emphasis on the client's confession of sin, which they recognize as cathartic. Subsequently, they mediate forgiveness through atonement, after clients confront their problems.

Techniques

Techniques used by Traditional Healers

The 1978 WHO Report stated that the methods and techniques traditional healers employ are somewhat closely-guarded secrets. Most of the techniques reviewed in this section were obtained through the efforts of patients and persistent field workers.

Levine and Padilla (1980) explained that therapists, witch doctors, spiritualists, or sorcerers all help their clients achieve comfort as they function in society. Each of these helpers establishes goals and employs techniques appropriate for his or her cultural milieu (Torrey, 1972). Traditional African healing processes are based on a conceptual scheme congruent with the client's worldview (Ìdòwú, 1985). Healing therefore allows clients to surrender their powers and assume roles prescribed by the healer.

The healers' roles are authoritative and their positions are reinforced by support from clients' family members and other interested parties. The interactions between healers and their clients differ because traditional

African healing is a community process that involves not only the client and the healer in individual therapy, but also the client's group and the mythical supernatural world.

The community-oriented process of healing raises the clients' expectancy of cure, helps them harmonize their inner conflicts, reintegrates them with their group and the spirit world, and stirs them up emotionally (Frank, 1978). In Africa, healing is generally geared towards complete personal integration into the cultural fabric; as a result, psychoanalysis and other insight-or behavior-oriented approaches, which focus on the individual, may be inappropriate. Rather, group counseling and other techniques that emphasize the clients' significant support groups and cultural identity seem more appropriate (Ìdòwú, 1985).

The Western counselor may see client's beliefs and the healer's techniques as "primitive" and non-scientific, but the positive outcomes demonstrate its potency. Effective counselors are those who can understand the inner and outer worlds of clients, interpret their emotional problems in terms of their worldview, and if possible, incorporate traditional beliefs in the process of undertaking the above (Ìdówú, 1985).

Mallum (1983) stated that the most common techniques used by Nigerian traditional healers are self-meditation by clients or their relatives, divination and incantation. The process of counseling used by traditional healers involves every gesture made by a client, followed by words or incantation mostly meaningful to the traditional healer alone (Mallum, 1983). Bulus (1989) enumerated the following techniques used by healers:

> Self-meditation by the client or relative; prayer to God or the gods; consultation of the traditional helper and the payment of fee where applicable; divination and incantation by using seeds up and down in specific styles, reading meaning from the face, using coins thrown in a small plate of water or looking at the palms of the hand to get meanings; before spelling out the action traditional healers want to take, (diagnosis comes after divination), when the secrets of the problem are made known to clients. The client is made to understand himself, his threats, liabilities or assets and told to use his opportunities through explanation, advice, and where necessary, persuasion to make sacrifice. Sacrifices could be using cereals, chickens, goats, or ducks, which are regarded as gifts to the gods to keep clients in harmony with the gods and used to give thanks and praises to the gods to have clients' problems solved. Psychotherapy is only used when there are serious problems which sacrifice and other positive social reinforcements cannot solve. Application of herbs and certain forces are used to relieve tension during this clinical treatment by traditional healers (pp. 109–110).

Ìdòwú (1985) provided examples of the four major categories of traditional healing techniques:

1. Activities, such as dances, rituals, confessions, and suggestions, constitute the first category. Individual participation in community activities, such as dances, rituals, and confessions release tension and promote communal mental health. Wallace (1970) referred to the above activities as therapeutically-effective control strategies. Diagnostic interviews and confessions in traditional healing include the therapeutic attributes of faith, suggestion, group support, and catharsis.
2. Traditional rituals performed at initiation ceremonies, include physical combat for strength, sex education for marriage, and initiation rites for those who will become healers help young people deal with anxieties and stressors associated with assuming adult responsibilities. These also serve preventive and developmental purposes.
3. Abreaction and catharsis, the third category of procedures, involves strategies for catharsis, temporarily indulging wishes or fantasies, and acting out a forbidden desire. These repressed impulses are allowed to be expressed, overtly or covertly, through rituals, meditation, or verbal therapy.
4. Milieu therapy, which constitutes the fourth category, allows clients to live with their families in a community, makes them part of the social system and reveals the richness that pervades in African culture (p. 84–85).

Traditional healing techniques, which result in certain environmental arrangements described above, take place within the traditional African culture and act as powerful buffers against social pressures and conflicts to promote good mental health.

Ambler (1994) discussed the efforts of "tribally" controlled colleges to integrate traditional American Indian techniques with Western medical colleges. This approach, according to him, will assist in promoting understanding of Indian traditional healing methods. Abas, Broadhead, Mbape, and Khumalo-Sakatukwa (1994) discovered that Zimbabwe training already incorporates and recognizes similar traditional healing processes. Zimbabwe, Swaziland and Nigeria medical administrators support integrating modern medical healing methods with traditional healing practices through the efforts of their respective National Associations of Traditional Healers and practicing Western medical experts.

Props and Cues

Clients consult traditional healers according to their perceived estimate of the healers' endowed supernatural powers. Props and cues are some of those tools that healers display to exhibit their supernatural powers. Props are part of the staging process in the presentation of self in a particular role (Davis, Boles, & Tatro, 1984).

Traditional healers' props include artifacts that demonstrate their expertise and authority. Healers use their knowledge and experience when selecting artifacts for their clients. Most props, which are handmade, are given to clients to be worn or used in different situations; some props are used as decorations in cars or homes or are worn on hands or necks (Davis, Boles and Tatro 1984).

Diviners' consulting rooms are said to be more elaborate than the stalls of market herbalists (Morris, 1986). Photographs, certificates from the healers' alma mater (which is usually from another older healer), several animal skins draped over the wall of the room, withered remains of owls or other animals, animal horns, or the skin of an enormous python are displayed in the traditional healers' consulting rooms. The floor may hold a large number of gourd containers and bottles containing a variety of root and bark infusions and oils containing wood ashes (Morris, 1986). Traditional healers use props and cues as sources of protection to bring about good health and blessings for their clients.

Healing Factors in Traditional Therapy

Healing can be accomplished through suggestions from traditional healers, ritual acts such as sacrifices, and alteration of the socio-physical and religious environment. Clients must implement the traditional healers' suggestion if they are to get well. Sacrifices are used to appease the gods to assist the clients to emerge from their predicament. Traditional healers look for and remove the socio-physical religious factors found to have caused the illness to alleviate their clients' sufferings and problems (Bulus, 1989).

The method of consultation is often determined by the seriousness of the clients' problems or sickness. For example, chronically ill and incapacitated clients, such as lepers and psychiatrically disabled clients, have to stay with the traditional healers until they are completely healed. These clients with serious diseases are accommodated in special treatment rooms in the practitioners' compound until they are declared to be well enough to go home (Ityavyar, 1987).

N'donazi(1991) depicted the healing wisdom, art, knowledge, and skills of traditional healers as unequaled, unparalleled and worthy of emulation. Root Bernstein believed that many discredited healing techniques and remedies of the past may yield fresh approaches to the treatment of cancer, heart disease, and infectious illnesses (McAuliffe, 1992).

Counseling and Western-Trained Nigerian Counselors

The present Western counseling theories and approaches studied in Western countries and currently in Nigerian Universities have their historical roots in Western religion, philosophy, ideas, and values (Saleh, 1989). Most Western-oriented counseling theories and approaches emphasize individualistic rather than collective family-oriented notions that are alien to non-Western cultures, such as Nigeria.

The field of counseling is exclusively monocultural because of the inordinate influence of Western culture (Saleh, 1989). Some of the contributors to and manifestations of this phenomenon are: (a) the deep historical and philosophical roots of counseling in Western culture, (b) the dominant theories, practice and approaches of counseling which make the assumption that counseling will take place within a Western culture, (c) the bulk of research and literature pertaining to counseling within the West, and (d) the emulation by non-Western nations of Western models of counseling (Saleh, 1989).

There exists the real danger that people who are instrumental in developing counseling within Nigeria could so over-adapt Western-based counseling techniques that they fail to perceive the importance of the need to develop models, techniques, and approaches appropriate to Nigerian culture. This may explain why many Nigerians, including well-educated ones, have more faith in traditional healers than in imported helpers (Saleh, 1989). Theories, models, research findings and techniques of application are not automatically transferable from a Western culture to a so-called traditional culture (Mar'i, 1982).

There is a need for the training programs of both Western and non-Western nations to be changed in such a way as to infuse the curriculum with counseling methods that reflect the different cultures that are represented there (Saleh, 1989). The profession of counseling needs to leave behind monoculturalism and become culturally reflective in order to allow counselors' roles to be shaped by the culture and circumstances in which they are working (Abonta, 1986).

Guidance and Counseling in Nigeria

Formal guidance programs were started in Nigeria towards the end of 1959 by Catholic Sisters at St Teresa's College in *Ìbàdàn* (Okon, 1983). A solid foundation was laid in the introduction of Western-based guidance and counseling practice in 1963 through the efforts of American educators at Comprehensive High School, in *Ayétòrò*, *Ògùn* State (Fáfúnwá, 1969).

The introduction of a new system of education referred to as the 6–3–3–4 educational system gave guidance and counseling a big boost in Nigeria (Adekson, 1987). This educational system, which mandates six years of elementary school education, three years of middle school education, three years of senior high school education, and four years of technical training, college or university education, also mandates guidance and counseling program in all the phases of education through a Federal Government White Paper (National Policy on Education, 1981). The involvement of the Federal Government in the introduction of guidance and counseling in schools paved the way for the first interaction between counselors and the public. Counselors had to deal with students, as well as their parents and family members in schools (Oláyínká, 1976 & Ìpàyẹ, 1986).

Recent research efforts have been geared mostly towards the improvement of traditional counseling in Nigeria (Ọláyínká, 1973 & Adekson, 1987). The Universities of *Ìlorin*, *Jos*, and Lagos, as well as Ọbáfémi Awólọ̀wọ̀ University at *Ilé-Ifẹ̀*, are greatly renowned for this approach and research undertaking (Bulus, 1989, Denga, 1983, Mallum, 1983, Mákindé, 1984, Achebe, 1986 & Adekson, 1987). These programs have allowed professors and graduate students to research new areas in traditional counseling. Six universities, *Jos*, *Ilé-Ifẹ̀*, *Ìbàdàn*, *Benin*, *Ìlọrin*, *Nsukka*, and Lagos, developed laudable but mostly Western-oriented programs, for the training of counselors at the graduate level (Adekson, 1987).

QUALITY AND CRITICISMS OF RESEARCH REVIEWED

In conclusion, the above summary reviewed primary research studies that utilized interview schedules, narrations, observations, case studies, and other qualitative methods. The review also summarized projects that combined quantitative and qualitative research methods.

Òjó (1967), Mbiti (1969), Mákindé (1973, 1974, 1978, 1980, 1984), Lámbò (1983), Mallum (1983), Salan and Maretzki (1983), Edwards (1983), Easthope (1986), Ìpàyẹ́ (1986), Mákindé (1987, 1988, 1995), Bulus (1989) and Saleh (1989) Ọdebíyì and Togonu-Bickersteth (1987), de Jong (1989), Veyrat & Ferrier (1989), Vontress (1991), Ezeji & Sarvela (1992), Agpeyong (1992), Rankin & Kappa (1993), MacLachlan (1993), Abas, Broadhead, Mbape & Khumalo-Sakatukwa (1994), Cassidy (1994) and Levers & Maki (1994 & 1995) gave first-hand information about their interactions with traditional healers in *Yorùbá* land, other parts of Nigeria, Africa, Malaysia, and other parts of the world. Epega & Neimark (1995) utilized first-hand narration to reveal the sacred facts of *Ifá* oracle.

Several researchers have described observations, interviews, and interactions with healers as first-hand accounts (Foster 1976; Ọdejídè et al. 1978; Rappaport 1980; Alonzo 1984; McCauley 1984; Torrey 1986; Nyamwaya 1987; Ngokwey 1988; Fabrega 1990; Witte 1991; Auge 1989; Ọdẹ́jídé et. al. 1989; Asuni 1990; Roder 1991; Hickson and Mokhobo 1992; N'donazi 1991; Schoepf 1992; Green 1992 and Levers & Maki 1994 & 1995). These scholars used qualitative methods to capture traditional healers' patterns of life, interactions with clients, and their modes of thought regarding the concept of illness and disease.

Ọdejídè, Ọlátawúrà, Sàndà & Oyènẹ́yẹ́ (1977) combined the use of surveys (quantitative) with interviews (qualitative) in their research on *Ìbàdàn* based Traditional Healers and mental health clients in *Yorùbá* land. Eskin (1989), Lepowsky (1990), and Murray and Shepherd (1993) combined the use of quantitative research methods with interviewing traditional healers. Foster (1976), Morris (1986), and Ngokwey (1988) combined the use of case-study approaches (qualitative) with interviewing (qualitative), and observations (qualitative) with active interactions with the healers they studied.

Other researchers, like Mákindé (1984), Mákindé (1988) and Epega & Neimark (1995), utilized historical analyses based on the latters' roles as diviners (*Ifá* priests) and close relationships with the healers they observed, lived and worked with, to highlight the functions and roles performed by Yorùbá Traditional Healers.

Most of the above researchers revealed their active involvement with traditional healers through the use of different qualitative research approaches. The different researchers' styles of interactions, interviewing, narrations and observations, coupled with the way they maintained their field notes, were useful to the present researcher.

SUMMARY

The literature reviewed in this chapter focused on traditional healers and discussed how healers' roles impact their clients. The major ethnic groups of Nigeria, *Yorùbá* and *Yorùbá* land were described as a prelude to the review. The roles, functions and techniques used by traditional healers all over the world and specifically by Yorùbá Traditional Healers were also reviewed to provide some insights into the ways in which culture affects the interactional relationships between healers and their clients. Issues such as myths and superstitions, herbalists' role and healing factors in traditional therapy were addressed to illustrate some of the underlying factors that affect healer-client relationships.

The literature revealed that clients become dependent on and have faith in traditional healers they consult because they are from the same culture. The literature also suggested that the culture in which people socialize determines the beliefs that they hold and the nature of their problems (Vontress, 1991). The way that clients perceive traditional healers' intervention as beneficial was also shown through the literature. The ethnomedical approach was reviewed to show how culturally-based beliefs about health and illness influence traditional healers' interactions with their clients.

I devoted attention to the herbalist's role in the review to show that traditional healers have varying roles. Healing factors in traditional therapy were discussed to reveal the underlying components of healers' functions and roles. Tradition was reviewed as an indirect source of knowledge transmitted from one generation to another.

I also described the functions and roles of traditional healers in an effort to show the importance of traditional healing in the world. Traditional healers were shown to have been as old as humanity, and the literature revealed that healers have been the source of care for many clients for centuries (Schusky & Culbert, 1967). The World Health Organization (1978) also reported that traditional medicine contributes to the health care of 80 percent of the world's population, including Nigeria where the majority of the rural population lacks access to Western-trained doctors, nurses, midwives and other paramedical health workers. Hence, the literature showed that traditional healers are the world's major source of available health care.

The literature further revealed that the techniques used by traditional healers vary from one culture to another and are intricately integrated into each society's cultural fabric. Self-meditation, prayers, divinations, incantations, reading meanings from the face, sacrifices, application of herbs, initiations, abreaction and catharsis, dances, rituals, using coins thrown into a small plate of water and reading the palms of the hand are some of the techniques used by traditional healers.

I also paid attention to closely related literature on the traditional systems of healing, general techniques used by healers and the roles and functions performed by traditional healers in the world. All traditional healers are confronted with the responsibilities of healing and solving their clients' problems within their respective cultural and environmental domains. The traditional healers closely interact with their clients as they perform these roles. The reviewed literature also alluded to the presence of Western- trained Nigerian counselors, and the prevalence of guidance and counseling in the country.

In total, I reported that culture plays an important part in the healing techniques that healers use, as traditional healers play important and expressive roles in all cultures in the world. Traditional healers devote a great deal of time and energy to interacting, helping, healing, curing, assisting, communicating with and relating to their clients.

Since the literature strongly supports conducting further research on the interpersonal techniques used by healers with their clients in different countries of the world, we specifically revisit these themes in the context of the Nigerian experience in Chapters Four and Five. In the meantime, additional literature on the use of, description of and justification for the case study methodology is provided in Chapter Three.

CHAPTER THREE
Methodology and Procedures

AS MENTIONED IN PRECEDING CHAPTERS, the goals of this volume are to understand what traditional healers do, discover what takes place between healers and their clients, recreate the practices, in-depth and unshared knowledge, and behaviors of seven Yorùbá Traditional Healers (YTHs) in their interactions with clients, and subsequently generate hypotheses regarding these interpersonal techniques. In furtherance of these aims, I observed, interacted with, videotaped and interviewed profiled healers during individual healing and group divining sessions with their clients, generated data from the information collected through the above methods, and derived hypotheses from these multiple sources of evidence (Yin, 1994).

Utilizing an exploratory case study approach allowed me to obtain first-hand information concerning YTHs' behavioral patterns, functions, roles and interactional relationships. In support of this enterprise, Ary, Jacobs and Razaviech (1979) asserted that the case study method provides an opportunity for researchers to heighten their insight into basic aspects of human behavior. Merriam (1988) also declared that "a qualitative case study is an intensive, holistic description and analysis of a bounded phenomenon such as a program, an institution, a person, a process or a social unit" (p. xii).

The discussion of the methods and procedures employed in this volume is subsumed under the following headings: setting and the language used for the research; support for the research; population and sample; description of the research subjects, the research entourage; the research instrument; descriptions of the procedures for data collection; interview schedule; observing, interviewing and videotaping Yorùbá healers; journal and record keeping; validity and reliability; data collection; approach to gathering and collecting the data; and summary.

The Case Study Methodology

The case study method allows the investigator to collect in-depth and extensive data on individuals' behavior (Miller and Warner, 1975). Merriam (1988) also agreed that case study approaches "concentrate attention on the way particular groups of people confront specific problems, taking a holistic view of the situation" (p.11). More specifically, by combining multiple sources of evidence, such as interviews and observations, also referred to as triangulation, I was able to enhance the benefits of the case study approach (Merriam, 1988; Denzin, 1970 and Yin, 1994).

As shown in Chapters Four and Five, this study developed hypotheses from its case facts rather than postulating them. In general, most case studies in the field of education are inductive, qualitative and hypothesis-generating, rather than quantitative and hypothesis-testing (Merriam, 1988). This inductive procedure enabled me to generate relevant and appropriate case facts, and investigate the interactional relationships between, and interpersonal techniques utilized by, Yorùbá Traditional Healers and their clients. Therefore, the case study's intensive nature allowed me to discover important and complex details relating to profiled individual(s) that might otherwise escape researchers (Kazdin, 1980, Yin 1994).

In the field of counseling, the case study approach to group research is very appropriate and fitting for research and evaluation (Chassan, 1967). When counselors and other investigators want to understand the causes of helpers and helpees' behaviors, they rely upon this method to collect extensive data relating to their studies (Miller & Warner, 1975; & Johnson, 1986). Furthermore, the use of the case study method in the investigation of traditional healers has provided scholars with detailed data pertaining to the activities of African healers. Nyamwaya (1987), among other authors, utilized the case study methodology to study indigenous healers in Kenya.

Similarly, the case study method provided the flexibility needed to observe and collect information on Yorùbá Traditional Healers' behaviors, their interactions with clients, attitudes, functions performed, services rendered to clients, and the interpersonal techniques used with clients. The method further assisted me in developing greater understanding of the dynamics of the healing culture and the healer-client relationship within the *Yorùbá* cultural domain.

Settings and the Language used for the Research

The four Southwestern states of *Ondó*, *Ògùn*, *Ọ̀yọ́* and *Ọ̀ṣun*, where members of the *Yorùbá* ethnic group predominantly reside, are the settings for this volume. This sub-region of Nigeria is very "natural and familiar" (Merriam 1988) to me. I was born in *Ọ̀yọ́* State, grew up in neighboring *Ọ̀ṣun* State, went to school and worked in all the four states covered by this study for several years. Fetterman's (1989) point that the researcher's interest is in understanding and describing a social and cultural scene from the "*emic*, or insider's perspective" (p. 12), was crucial in the design of this study. Throughout this project, I give an insider's perspective of what Yorùbá Traditional Healers do as a member of the *Yorùbá* ethnic group.

Yorùbá is the official language used by the healers in everyday transactions with their clients (See *Yorùbá* questions in Appendix B). Although dialects vary within and between *Yorùbá* states, all profiled Traditional Healers in each of the four states where the study was undertaken understand the basic *Yorùbá* language. Owing to my understanding and prior knowledge of different *Yorùbá* dialects, I surmounted communication problems that otherwise would have impeded this project.

Support for the Research

I consulted elders, wise men and the following experts: Professor Olú Mákindé, formerly of the Counseling Department and the Dean of the Faculty of Education, at the *Ilé-Ifẹ̀*-based Obáfẹ́mi Awólọ́wọ̀ University (OAU), Nigeria; Professor M. Akin Mákindé, the Chair of OAU's Philosophy Department in 1994; and Professor Akínṣọlá Akìwọwọ, former Chair of OAU's Department of Sociology and Anthropology.

These consultants have conducted extensive research on traditional healers and different ethnic groups in Nigeria. Also, these professors have lived, worked, consulted, and interacted with YTHs. Professor Akin Mákindé is a YTH's son and an ardent researcher in this field; one of his studies on traditional healers was published by Ohio University in 1988. As a researcher, Professor Olú Mákindé has undertaken over 30 years of research with YTHs. For his part, Professor Akínṣọla Akìwọwọ spent over 30 years researching different aspects of Yorùbá traditional healing, and was an apprentice to Chief *Odikun* of *Ondó* town in Nigeria. In order to enrich this venture, I also solicited the assistance of Deans of healers, elders, community leaders, and paraprofessionals who work with traditional healers in different ways in *Yorùbá* land.

Population and Sample

I studied seven Yorùbá Traditional Healers who included four herbalists (*oníṣègùn/adábunṣe*): one each, from *Ọ̀yó*, *Ọ̀ṣun*, *Ondó*, and *Ògùn* States, and three diviners *(Ifá priests)*. The four herbalists, Drs. Awótáyọ̀, Akínọlá, Adésànyà and Chief Abíọ́lá, were chosen from the above four states where over 50 percent of *Yorùbá* live.

Additionally, I was advised by Professor M. Akin Mákindé to interview Chief Awórẹ́ni, an *Ifá* Priest (diviner), and also observe the functions of Chiefs Awórẹ́ni, Awójọbí, and Ọlájídé, the three *Ifá* Priests (Diviners) working together in group divining in one session. The addition of three diviners to this research allowed the depiction of the totality of what is known as traditional medicine among the *Yorùbá* (Mákindé, 1994, Appendix A). Traditional medicine in *Yorùbá* land "consists of the practices of *Onísègùn/Adáhunṣe* (herbalists); and *Ifá priests* (diviners)" (Mákindé, 1994, Appendix A). Information concerning the differences and similarities between the interactions of herbalists and diviners is outlined in detail in Appendix A.

Only four notable and experienced herbalists (*oníṣègùn*), and three diviners (Ifá priests), the two groups generically referred to as *babaláwo* in this study, were profiled and videotaped; due to time constraints, four herbalists and the chief diviner were interviewed. I employed "purposeful sampling" (Chein 1981, p. 440), which is the deliberate selection of multiple cases for the purposes of discovering, understanding and gaining new insights regarding the activities of traditional healers.

Selected Yorùbá Traditional Healers and diviners were at least 50 years old and had at least 10 years experience in the practice of traditional healing. The age of Yorùbá Traditional Healers is of importance to this study because its accompanying prestige, status, experience, and reputation are synonymous with respect and wisdom in *Yorùbá* land (Òjó, 1967). The seven selected healers and diviners command great respect and prestige in the community as evidenced by their personal involvement and leadership roles within their community, *Yorùbá*, Nigerian and African Traditional Healing circles. Their personal involvement and leadership roles are revealed in the results presented in the next two chapters.

These seven Yorùbá Traditional Healers were chosen based on feedback from *Yorùbá* kings, chiefs, elders, Dean of healers, community members who have interacted with the chosen healers as clients and confidants; from other Yorùbá Traditional Healers; and from Professors M. Akin Mákindé, Olú Mákindé and Akínsoṣlá Akìwọwọ, who have all done extensive research on Yorùbá Traditional Healers.

Moreover, the choice was based on feedback about the healers' active involvement as leaders within African, Nigerian and Yorùbá Traditional Healing Associations. Feedback from professors at *Ògùn*, *Ọ̀yọ́*, and *Ondó* State universities, community experts, some of the seven healers' former clients, and Chiefs in *Ilé-Ifẹ̀*, *Ìjèbú Igbó*, *Ẹrìn Ìjèṣà* and *Ìbàdàn* were also helpful in identifying appropriate Yorùbá Traditional Healers. I further interviewed chiefs, community elders and other individuals in the marketplace of the healers' towns and villages of *Ìbàdàn*, *Ilé-Ifẹ̀*, *Ẹrìn Ìjèṣà* and *Ìjèbú Igbó*, and talked to at least four other healers in each of these cities and villages to further identify the subjects for this study.

Final selection was based on age, years of experience, number of years that healers spent on internship before becoming healers, recommendations of my three consultants and those of the Dean of healers who recommended the best healer in each state based on prior interactions with them, their reputations and the criteria discussed above. For instance, Chief Abíọ̀lá (Herbalist/*Oníṣègùn* 3), one of the Yorùbá Traditional Healers recommended for this study, was one of the subjects in Professor Akin Mákindé's 1988 study. The professor is also familiar with the divining activities of the three diviners, because of his other research efforts and position within Ọbáfémi Awólọwọ̀ University's Philosophy Department.

Lastly, I chose seven all male Yorùbá Traditional Healers (four herbalists and three diviners) for this study because, traditionally, *babaláwo* have been mostly men in *Yorùbá* land. Female Yorùbá Traditional Healers were excluded from this study to ensure unanimity and uniformity.

DESCRIPTION OF THE RESEARCH SUBJECTS

Babaláwo, referred to as herbalists or medicine men, and comprising of *four Oníṣègùn* (herbalists) and *three Ifá priests* (diviners), were the seven Yorùbá Traditional Healers examined in this study. *Babaláwo* attend promptly to all of the needs brought to them for healing by their mostly-*Yorùbá* clients. People who are in trouble are invited for counseling and one-to-one interactions with the *babaláwo* (Mákindé, 1974).

Babaláwo prescribe herbs and medicines which are made from the roots of various plants, believed to possess the ability to cure a variety of problems such as infertility, mental disorders, bad omens, impotence, and fractures (Cowan, 1987), and also are respected members of their communities. By virtue of this last role, *babaláwo* have become the 'listening ears' for families, individuals, and people in distress. For this reason, Nigerians from all walks of life seek the expertise of these knowledgeable ones. The examined four herbalists (*Oníṣègùn*) include Drs. Awótáyọ̀, Akínọlá, Adésànyà and Chief Abíọ́lá, while the diviners (*Ifá* priests) include Chiefs Awórẹ́ni, Awójọbí and Ọlájídé.

Dr. Awótáyọ̀ was born in 1921 in *Ẹrìn Ìjẹ̀ṣà, Ọ̀ṣun* State. He was reared as a Christian in the Apostolic Church, resided in *Ẹrìn Ìjẹ̀ṣà* and inherited traditional healing and farming from his grandfather, Akínláyẹmí, who was a hunter, farmer, healer and blacksmith. Dr. Awótáyọ̀, who never had formal Western educational training, obtained his healing power through heredity (*àjogúnbá*) and has been in traditional healing practice for over 47 years. He sharpened his healing power through observations, fasting and incessant prayers to God Almighty (*Olódùmarè*). Dr. Awótáyọ̀ specializes in treating clients with "brain disorders" (*àrùn ọpọlọ*). He is presently married to many wives and has several children, one of whom became a healer under his tutelage.

Dr. Akínọlá, a professional chartered accountant, was born in *Ìbàdàn*, the *Ọ̀yọ́* State capital, in 1935. Dr. Akínọlá resides at *Ọlọ́gẹ̀dẹ̀* a suburb of *Ìbàdàn*, and he, like Dr. Awótáyọ̀, inherited his healing power from his father, a renowned *Ìbàdàn* Traditional Healer. Dr. Akínọlá comes from a line of traditional healers, with his grandfather also being a reputable healer in *Ìbàdàn* and its environs. He has been in the healing practice for 30 years and specializes in general traditional healing and making, mixing, dispensing and selling locally-prepared herbs. Dr. Akínọlá, who is a devout Moslem, is an *Alhaji* by virtue of his pilgrimage to Mecca, and is married with seven children.

Chief Abíọ́lá of Abíọ́lá Native Hospital was born around 1910 and resided in *Ayégúnlẹ̀ Èkìtì* in *Ondó* State in 1994. He was, as of 1994, the *Eisikin* (a Chieftaincy title) of *Ayégúnlẹ̀ Èkìtì*. He was born and raised there, and later moved to *Ìbàdàn*, where he worked as a clerk for many years before retiring to practice traditional healing in his hometown. Chief Abíọ́lá obtained his healing power through training as an apprentice to his uncle and an intern to other experts in *Ondó* State. Prior to this time, his maternal uncle had identified his innate knowledge of herbs and healing when he was very young.

The chief, who never attended a formal Western school, was self taught in the knowledge and practice of traditional healing. Chief Abíọ́lá has been in the healing practice for over 52 years, and he specializes in obstetrics and gynecology. Chief Abíọ́lá, like Dr. Awótáyọ̀, is a well-known farmer in addition to being a healer. The chief, who has many wives and children, trained one of his sons as a traditional healer.

Dr. Adésànyà, the owner of Àláfíá Táyọ Pharmacy and Herbal Home, is a traditional healer who was born in *Ìjẹ̀bú Igbó*, *Ògùn* State, in 1909. Like Drs. Akinọlá and Awótáyọ̀, he also received his power through heredity and natural endowments. Dr. Adésànyà inherited, observed and learned healing methods from his father, and has practiced traditional healing for over 60 years. His area of expertise is general healing, mixing and dispensing herbs, and curing blood-borne diseases. Dr. Adésànyà, who was raised in the Anglican Church as a Christian, has many wives and children. Whilst the doctor regretted that none of his children were interested in learning the methods of traditional healing, one of his grandchildren has currently shown some interest in the profession.

Chief Awóreni, the only profiled chief diviner, is the *Àràbà* of *Ilé-Ifẹ̀* and the *Oníṣesìn Àgbáyé* (the highest *Ifá* Priest in the world). Born in 1932, in *Ilé-Ifẹ̀*, *Ọ̀ṣun* State, Chief Awóreni inherited his divining power from his paternal grandfather who was renowned for using his divining power to resurrect the dead, and from instructions from supernatural beings. Chief Awóreni, who never had a Western-oriented education, learned mechanical engineering as a vocation. He has divined for over 22 years, has many wives and children, and has taught two of his younger children the intricacies of divining.

Chief Awójọbí was born in *Ilé-Ifẹ̀* in 1922. He is also a priest and the *Aféódigba* of *Ilé-Ifẹ̀* city. The chief, who lived in *Ilé-Ifẹ̀* most of his life, is one of the three diviners, along with Chiefs Awórẹ́ni and Awójọbí, in charge of making sacrifices for the city and for *Yorùbá* land. In addition to performing divining rites, Chief Awójọbí is a farmer, married to many wives and has several children.

Chief Ọlájídé, the *Olórí Awo* of *Ilé-Ifẹ̀* was born in *Ilé-Ifẹ̀* in 1921 and has spent the majority of his life there. He is also a farmer, and like the above-named diviners, is experienced in handling problems linked to supernatural causations. The Chief, who was never trained in a Western-oriented school, practices traditional religion, like Chiefs Awóréni and Awójọbí, and has several wives and children.

Prior to undertaking interviews with and observations of the aforementioned Yorùbá Traditional Healers, I informed them of this study's purpose and methods (see introduction to the Interview Schedule in Appendix B & C). Following from this presentation, the healers all verbally agreed to participate in the study to enhance research efforts on traditional healing. I provided the time and opportunity for each healer to ask questions and express comments concerning the nature and aims of this project. I further assured the seven healers that all information gathered for this study would be used solely for the research purposes for which it was intended.

THE RESEARCH ENTOURAGE

The fact that the researcher's father is a *Yorùbá* elder closely acquainted with Yorùbá Traditional Healers in *Ilé-Ifẹ̀* and *Iléṣà* (both in *Ọ̀ṣun* State), made my trips for this study a successful one. My father was one of the important members of the entourage who visited and studied all the Yorùbá Traditional Healers with me. His presence was an added advantage to this research because of his advanced age, which is synonymous with wisdom among the *Yorùbá*, and because of his past contacts and relationships with *Yorùbá* Healers.

The driver, who grew up in *Ilé-Ifẹ̀* , is both a strong believer in traditional medicine and healing, and a regular client of Yorùbá Traditional Healers. Kúnlé, the videotape expert who recorded all the activities with profiled healers, possessed personal experiences with traditional healers. His work as a professional recorder had taken him to several *Yorùbá* cities and villages where he taped traditional activities for Kings, Chiefs and important dignitaries. In sum, the fact that members of the research entourage have experience with traditional healers not only aided me in collecting relevant data, but also made the results more authentic and rich.

TOOLS FOR DATA COLLECTION

As mentioned in prior discussions, I was born in *Ọ̀yọ́* State, grew up, went to school and worked as a teacher, a school counselor, a vice principal, acting principal and educational administrator for a number of years in different *Yorùbá* towns. According to Merriam (1988), data is mediated through the researcher rather than through some inanimate inventory such as the questionnaire. Furthermore, Guba and Lincoln (1981), opined that: "in situations where motives, attitudes, beliefs, and values direct much, if not most of human activity, the most sophisticated instrumentation we possess is still the careful observer, the human being who can watch, see, listen, question, probe, and finally analyze and organize his direct experience" (p. 213). Serving as both the researcher and primary data collector therefore allowed healers to respond directly and positively to my inquiries. In so doing, existing knowledge regarding Yorùbá Traditional Healers' cultural milieu and nonverbal interactions will be expanded.

Description of the Procedures for Data Collection

Several data collection strategies were used for collecting data with Yorùbá Traditional Healers. These strategies included *self-prepared, semi-structured interviews*; *participant observations*; *journals*; and *videotaping*. I prepared structured interviews in *Yorùbá* Language and translated them into English Language (Appendices B & C) to elicit information from four herbalists and the chief diviner about their personal lives, experiences and lives as healers. I utilized basic knowledge of the case study approach to collect data with the help of the videotape recorder.

By investigating Yorùbá Traditional Healers, this volume seeks to discover their roles and functions, behaviors, interactional relationships and personal characteristics and communication in relation to their clients. I employed several procedures, described in turn below, to capture the essence and details of healer-client interactions in the most in-depth and inclusive manner possible.

Interview Schedule

I obtained information from traditional healers through the use of self-prepared, semi-structured interviews (Appendices B & C). This interview schedule asked a set of questions to explore issues related to the interpersonal techniques used by selected traditional healers.

The elicited answers helped me to learn about and understand the variables that are commonly attributed to individuals who are healers among the *Yorùbá*. Elsewhere, similar sets of questions have yielded valuable information regarding the interactions of Malaysian healers with their clients (Salan and Maretzki, 1983). Consequently, the interview schedules for this volume were constructed by using a structure similar to that described by Salan and Maretzki (1983), and reflective of studies conducted by Mákindé (1974), Mákindé (1988) and Vontress (1991).

The interview schedule was reviewed by Professors M. Akin Mákindé, Akínṣọlá Akìwọwọ and Olú Mákindé, this study's three research field consultants, before it was employed in the data collection process. The use of the interview schedule enabled me to perceive and capture a broader view of the world of Yorùbá Traditional Healers as a group.

An interview generally engenders the development of a total picture of the individual(s) under consideration (Watson, 1963). Relatedly, Patton

(1980) explained that people are interviewed to identify feelings, thoughts, intentions and other variables that they cannot directly observe. Interviewing therefore allowed me to enter into the traditional healers' world from their own perspectives, while enabling Yorùbá Traditional Healers to freely express their inner thoughts. Hence, Watson (1963) argued that one of the advantages of directed interview is that "it ensures that all questions considered relevant to the issue at hand are answered in some fashion" (p.86). He further stated that interview schedules provide a modicum of flexibility.

I posed questions based on the five Yorùbá Traditional Healers' (four herbalists and the chief diviner) backgrounds and demographic characteristics to identify the traditional healers' social position and status in the community (Appendices B & C). Questions about their age, level of education, ethnic group, residence/mobility, number of years in training, gender, marital status, other occupation besides healing, period of apprenticeship, cost of services, types of clientele, source of healing power (e.g., inherited, supernaturally endowed, initiation rituals, or dream-invoked), were asked. Questions that revealed information about healers' relevant life experiences prior to entering the profession were also asked. The answers gave me some insight into the YTHs' personalities and their individual characteristics as unique members within the *Yorùbá* community (Table 1).

Affective questions were designed to discover what the traditional healers feelings were toward their clients when they came in for healing. These provided an understanding of traditional healers' experiences, thoughts and responses, and how traditional healers' feelings affect their interactions with clients. Additionally, *Knowledge* questions were asked to discover what traditional healers perceive as factual information regarding their functions and roles in their healing relationships with clients.

Overall, the goal of these questions was to "develop pertinent hypotheses and propositions for further inquiry" (Yin, 1994, p. 5). Consequently, I chose *Yorùbá* words, with which the traditional healers were all familiar, as the mode of questioning (See Appendix B for interview guide). Since I am conversant with the *Yorùbá* Language, I printed the questions and the English Language translation (Appendices B & C), and transcribed the *Yorùbá* responses from the interviewing process and the videotaped sessions into English Language.

Professors Akin Mákindé, Akínṣọlá Akìwọwọ, and Olú Mákindé, the researcher's field consultants who are also very fluent in *Yorùbá* and English, examined and approved the translations. Mrs. Tokunbo Adekambi, a *Yorùbá* Language Lecturer at Howard University's Department of Modern Languages in Washington D. C. in 1996, also examined and approved the translation from *Yorùbá* to English Language, and placed accent marks on all the *Yorùbá* words used in this study.

Words denoting respect were chosen to extract information from the healers, as respect for elders is part of the unwritten norms in *Yorùbá* culture (Òjó, 1967). I therefore used respectful words and gestures while interacting with *Yorùbá* Traditional Healers referenced throughout this volume.

Videotaping Yorùbá Traditional Healers

The videotaping of seven Yorùbá Traditional Healers' interactions with their clients during actual sessions was one of the tools used in this project to collect data. As previously noted, the case study inquiry "relies on multiple sources of evidence" (Yin, 1994, p.13), which for the purposes of this study, included a combination of videotaping, interviewing, and observations.

Specifically, videotaping, which captured the interpersonal techniques that healers used with their clients, was undertaken by Kúnlé in the clinics and compounds of four herbalists and three diviners. Interviews and interactional activities of each of the four herbalists with five clients were videotaped for five days. Videotaping the interview took the first day in each traditional healer's home.

During the remaining four days, I videotaped, observed and recorded the healers' interactions with their clients in the formers' homes, compounds, clinics and hospitals. I also spent one day interviewing Chief Awóreni, the *Àràbà* (*Oníşèsìn Àgbáyé*) and the chief diviner. The last two days were spent videotaping, observing, and recording the three diviners' interactions with their clients. The videotaping of all the sessions, plus the observations, interactions and interviews with the seven YTHs, took 31 days altogether.

I discovered that the presence of the video camera and other taping equipment did not affect the outcome of the healers' interactions or the methods or techniques they used with their clients. A review of the tapes, and anecdotal feedback from my field consultants and from elders in the community who have consulted traditional healers on numerous occasions, confirmed the researcher's observation regarding the non-intrusive nature of taped recordings.

Observing Yorùbá Traditional Healers

In order to observe a wide range of activities and gain detailed firsthand knowledge of what was occurring in the healers' clinics, homes, or hospitals, I compiled relevant information using the participant observation method. I spent five days on site with each of the four traditional healers observing client sessions with the healers. This resulted in five visits to each of the four herbalist's compound for five consecutive days to complete this process. There was a three-day visit to the chief diviner's compound to observe the three diviners' activities.

The average time spent per day was eight hours. During the participant observation periods, the Yorùbá Traditional Healers conducted their daily healing functions and roles while I observed the healers' interactions with their clients, family members and other community members. This allowed me to gain a broader understanding of the healers' affective world and the nature of their relationships with clients, family members and the larger community.

I took mental and observational notes of the behaviors (verbal and nonverbal) of each Yorùbá Traditional Healer to enhance the study's value. These mental notes were later transcribed into written reflections and accounts of all traditional healers' behaviors in my journal. I utilized observation, in addition to interviewing and videotaping, to capture any nonverbal information that was left out of the note-taking process. This is in line with Merriam's (1988) contention that "observations differ from interviews in that the researcher obtains a firsthand account of the phenomenon of interest rather than relying on someone else's interpretation" (p. xii). This volume purposely employed direct observation to understand the behaviors, communication patterns, interactional and interpersonal relationships, and feeling states of each of the studied Yorùbá Traditional Healers, as well as the group as a whole. Scheduled and semi-structured interviews, and videotaping were used in conjunction with direct observation to deepen the understanding of the healing culture and structure.

Guba and Lincoln (1981) contended that "... in situations where motives, attitudes, beliefs, and values direct much, if not most of human activity, the most sophisticated instrumentation we possess is still the careful observer—the human being who can watch, see, listen ... question, probe, and finally analyze and organize his direct experience" (p. 213). Therefore, observations allowed me to enter into the "here and now" framework of the YTHs studied. As such, the participant observer methodology provided me with an excellent view of the subject(s)'or person's world (Bruyn 1966).

Observation as a research procedure was utilized from my very first contact with Dr. Awótáyọ̀ the first traditional healer and through subsequent interactions with the other healers. I observed how the healers talked to their clients, related to them during healing sessions, responded to clients' questions about being healed, and performed their healing functions, as well as healers' tone and speed of speech. Evidence and description of all sequences of events, which occurred during interactions among healers and clients, were also noted. Moreover, I observed non-verbal communications such as eye contact, body movements, touching, smiles and different gestures, such as hugs and respectful gestures, between clients and healers.

As amply demonstrated in Chapters Four and Five, I observed that the profiled herbalists, Drs. Awótáyọ̀, Akínọlá, Adésànyà and Chief Abíọ́lá, allowed clients to freely explain their problems before diagnosing and suggesting remedies to them. On the other hand, Chiefs Awóreni, Awójọbí and Ọlájídé went into the divining mode to find out the nature of the problem from *Ifá* before asking clients any question. These and related observations strengthened the interview results.

In line with the aforementioned fact, Sundberg (1977) stated that observations and interviews supplement each other, and noted that we employ the former in everyday life in our effort to understand other people. Observation as a tool for collecting data is extremely beneficial in developing a broader, extensive and comprehensive investigation of the techniques, behaviors, functions, and interactions of Yorùbá Traditional Healers, and identifying, examining, evaluating, and explaining the constitution of their healing culture.

Journal and Record Keeping

My record keeping procedures involved maintaining a file which consisted of the following: a research journal, interview field notes, questions from my observations during the field study, transcripts from interviews conducted in *Yorùbá* (Appendices B & C), and reports of feedback from field consultants. I collected and kept important and relevant research and field notes as a way of capturing the full observation of interpersonal techniques used by YTHs.

During the course of research, journals were kept to enhance the comprehensiveness of collected information. The journal keeping procedure allowed me to collect data on the seven YTHs in their natural environment. Barker (1968) supports the use of the ecological model to examine human behavior because it is the most appropriate tool for capturing the healers' whole environment. Barker (1968) and Sundberg (1977) further concurred that the surroundings and environmental forces of individuals impinge significantly on their well-being and existence. Consequently, I recorded quotes, paraphrases, and summaries of conversations in *Yorùbá*, and translated them into English after they were verified as accurate by my consultants. I also recorded individual characteristics, such as age, level of formal education, level of interactions, nonverbal behavior, and physical surroundings.

My field notes for this study went beyond simply including tentative interpretations of what the data meant, to including my reactions to the data. The actual behaviors and tones of Yorùbá Traditional Healers were recorded in an attempt to remain objective. Field notes were recorded during and after my observations of the healers' interactions and healing relationships with clients. More extensive notes were written each night, immediately after leaving the healers' clinics, homes or hospitals. Equally, physical and personal clues were objectively and daily recorded in my field notes. This review, which consisted of different notes written on each healer, provided data that I could not have discovered through interviewing alone.

The field notes for this research comprehensively included identifying information such as the date, time, setting and subjects of videotaping and observation. I also recorded all the nonverbal interactions in the form of gestures, eye contact and interactional relationships, as seen through interviewing and recorded through videotaping. The observational field notes and interview schedule notes were typewritten at the end of each day. Finally, I assembled the notes, which became part of the case facts, at the end of the 31 days of research, and translated the *Yorùbá* Language transcripts. The translations were subsequently examined by Professors Olú Mákindé, Akin Mákindé, Akìwọwọ and Mrs. Adékàmbí for accuracy.

VALIDITY AND RELIABILITY

Validity and reliability are of major concern in case study research because every researcher needs to conduct and contribute knowledge that is believable and trustworthy. Construct validity, "establishing correct operational measures for the concepts being studied" (Yin, 1994, p.33), was guaranteed in this volume through the use of triangulation or multiple sources of evidence. This strategy improves the quality and richness of data, as well as the accuracy of case study findings.

In particular, this richness is shown through testing one source of information against another or with another to improve findings, offer an explanation, or prove a hypothesis: "The rationale for this strategy is that the flaws of one method are often the strengths of another, and by combining methods, observers can achieve the best of each, while overcoming their unique deficiencies" (Denzin, 1970, p. 308).

Reliability refers to the extent to which one's findings can be replicated. I consulted with Professors Akin Mákindé, Olú Mákindé and Akínṣọlá Akìwọwọ regarding my research undertaking, as well as my reactions to the taped recordings and healers' activities. This consultation allowed me to check the accuracy of these reactions, obtain necessary feedback and review the taped recordings of the sessions after interviewing and observing the healers. These experts' critical feedback regarding my research vis-à-vis their past experiences with the population also strengthened this study's reliability. Merriam (1988) referred to this last method of consultation as peer examination, that is, "asking colleagues to comment on the findings as they emerge" (p. 169).

I also asked the healers, my parents, who watched the videotaped sessions with me during the daily reviews and the clients seen by the healers for feedback at the end of each taped session. I solicited these individuals' feedback on techniques, the healers' mode of interaction with their clients, the functions that healers performed and other culturally relevant matters. This extensive consultation helped, by means of a variety of sources, to reduce artificial responses and increase the study's validity (Merriam, 1988). In broad terms, establishing chains of evidence and having key informants review the drafts of the case study reports also strengthen construct validity (Yin, 1994).

In total, I spent 31 days conducting on-site observations, videotaping and interviewing traditional healers and the diviners. Spending this length of time with the healers allowed me to fully observe and understand the traditional healers, and thereby increased this project's validity and reliability.

Data Collection

This work incorporated several data collection methods in my quest to investigate the seven Yorùbá Traditional Healers studied. Before the data collection process was performed, I informed the seven Yorùbá Traditional Healers about the purpose of the study and its objectives, and explained the reason for the use of different data gathering procedures. The seven subjects were all informed of my interests and the purpose of conducting and pursuing research on YTHs with their clients.

I informed all the Yorùbá Traditional Healers of the need to investigate the total dynamics of their actions, which included the interactional relationships between their clients and themselves, their behaviors, functions and roles, approaches, methods and techniques and how culture influenced their interactions. My intention, as well as those of my consultants and the healers themselves, was to enhance the understanding of the healing relationship. It was also expected that the data collected from this undertaking would permit helping professionals to address the needs of traditional healers.

As the main investigator, I collected all data using interview schedules, journal keeping records, participant observation, physical evidence and videotaping. In collecting data through the use of the interview schedule, I utilized videotapes to obtain the subjects' verbal and non-verbal responses. This method was used to enhance and magnify the intensity and authenticity of the data collection. In line with this objective, Barker (1968) stated that observation is an effective technique that can be used to understand and study the human organism in its natural environment. He added that the direct observation of human subjects in their natural environment limits the distortion of the observed behavior. Similarly, Watson (1963) contended that the structured interview provides the researcher with the ability to control the direction of the interview, while the semi-structured interview "permits expression of the desired information and at the same time allows the conversation to find its own paths with a minimum of direction" (p.87).

Approach to Gathering and Presenting the Data

In preparing for the presentation of all data collected from this intensive, in-depth and inductive investigation of the interpersonal techniques used by Yorùbá Traditional Healers, I assessed individual healers and their clients. This was accomplished by considering cultural factors relating to both parties (Saleh, 1986; Pedersen & Pedersen, 1989; Tylor, 1989; Vontress, 1991; Ezeji & Sarvela, 1992 and Ìdòwú, 1985).

The investigation of the behavior utilized by Yorùbá Traditional Healers with their clients was done in conjunction with an examination of the subject's physical, private or personal worlds (Binswanger, 1962). This approach to data collection and review particularly combined the approaches of Binswanger (1962), Esen (1972), Fábùnmi (1975), Gardner (1964), Johnson (1986), Kleinman (1980), Lámbò (1983), Levers & Maki (1995), Mákindé (1988), Mákindé (1974), Mallum (1983), Ngokwey (1968), Nyamwaya (1987), Oyèbọ̀lá (1980) and Vontress (1991), to heighten the comprehensiveness of this volume's investigation of the entire group of Yorùbá Traditional Healers. Thus, I collected data on healers as a whole person (a personalized approach), emphasizing the healers' interrelational and interactional functions with their clients. This approach of data collection provided the foundation for generating data and formulating hypotheses on Yorùbá Traditional Healers.

In addition, I used the case data collected from the journal keeping records, observations, interview schedule and semi-structured interviews, and from the videotaped recordings, to reflect the interpersonal, physical, psychological and spiritual worlds of Yorùbá Traditional Healers. Information on the interactional-interrelational functions performed by Yorùbá Traditional Healers vis-à-vis their clients was gathered from the videotaped sessions, in conjunction with the interview schedule, semi-structured interviews, impressionist observations, and journal keeping records to enhance the validity of this case study's hypotheses.

Summary

This chapter outlined the methods and procedures used in this volume. My discussion specifically described the multidimensional procedure utilized to generate the hypotheses derived from obtained results. In developing a comprehensive approach to the examination and understanding of examined YTHs, the physical, interpersonal and private or personal worlds of each Yorùbá Traditional Healer were incorporated into this study's research design to augment the intensiveness and depth of this investigation (Binswanger, 1962).

As shown in ensuing analyses, this volume examined and addressed the interactional-interrelational dimensions of YTHs' dealings with their clients, to intensify the value and validity of the data collected. The work utilized several approaches: interviewing individual Yorùbá Traditional Healers through the use of interview schedule and semi-structured interviews; participant observation; researcher's interactions with the healers in their homes, clinics or hospitals; journal keeping and videotaping to enhance the scope and richness of all data collected.

I collected data using the above methods and procedures to reflect the Yorùbá Traditional Healers' interpersonal techniques, personality characteristics and behaviors toward their clients. The case study method enabled me to interact directly with the Yorùbá Traditional Healers in their natural cultural environment. This also contributed to my discovery of the wide array of information relating to the interpersonal techniques used by each healer.

The hypotheses delineated in Chapters Four and Five were generated from the data derived from the case by case description of daily activities of Yorùbá Traditional Healers. Responses to questions in the Interview Schedule in Appendix B (translated in Appendix C) contributed to my comprehensive understanding of Yorùbá Traditional Healers' relationships with their clients. This understanding was enhanced through my use of observations, interactions, interviewing, videotaping and reviewing videotaped sessions and field notes.

The conclusion that Yorùbá Traditional Healers' behaviors stem from having a similar culture with their clients was traced to subjects' responses, which are presented in later chapters. Analyses of my observations, Yorùbá Traditional Healers' responses and the results of their interactions with their clients are discussed in Chapters IV and V under "Case Facts and Hypotheses."

CHAPTER FOUR

Case Facts and Hypotheses

CHAPTERS FOUR AND FIVE PRESENT RESULTS AND HYPOTHESES related to the interpersonal techniques used by seven Yorùbá Traditional Healers of Nigeria. To realize these goals, this intensive case study assesses the relationship between seven Yorùbá Healers and their clients. I interviewed and/or observed seven male Yorùbá Traditional Healers; four herbalists, Drs. Awótáyọ̀, Akínọlá, Adésànyà and Chief Abíọ́lá, were 73, 62, 85 and 84 years old respectively in 1994, and three diviners, Chiefs Awóreni (the Àràbà), Awójọbí and Ọlájídé were 62, 72 and 73 years old respectively during the same period.

By employing a case study methodology and participant observation approach, I derived hypotheses from an investigation into the nature of Yorùbá Traditional Healers' physical, interpersonal, and private or personal worlds, their daily activities and experiences, and interactions with their clients within diverse healing environments. This critical examination of the interpersonal techniques used by Yorùbá Traditional Healers was undertaken through participant observation (via hospital, home or clinic visits), videotapes, scheduled interviews and journal records.

Responses to interview questions analyzed in later sections refer to both *Yorùbá* questions in Appendix B and to the English translation in Appendix C of the Interview Schedules. Profiled traditional healers responded to the questions listed in Appendix B with *Yorùbá* words. Consequently, I quoted some of the healers' exact words in *Yoruba* and subsequently offered the English translations throughout Chapters Four and Five. Questions and certain answers were also written in English using quotation marks to ensure easier readability. Tables 1 and 2 at the end of the book portray the "Healer Characteristics" and "Healer Support for Hypotheses" generated in this section.

Specifically, this volume examined healers' worlds, life patterns and experiences as a unit or body. This procedure was utilized by focusing on the communication (verbal and nonverbal) and interactional behaviors affecting clients' and healers' personal and physical worlds within the *Yorùbá* healing environment, healer-client relationships, individual healer's treatment strategies, diviner-client relationships, diviners' treatment strategies, diagnoses in healing and divining, healing interventions and encounters, and healing techniques. As Bruyn (1966) stated, the participant observer in his scientific role "seeks to apprehend, register, interpret, and conceptualize the social facts and meanings which he finds in a prescribed area of study" (p.18). In the next section, I focus on the background and status of Yorùbá Traditional Healers. This information was garnered by posing the questions in Appendix B to the profiled healers.

Yorùbá Traditional Healers' (YTHS') Background and Status

I posed the following question to the seven healers: "Do you perform other duties/work in addition to divining/healing?" The responses of *babaláwo's*, which are captured by Dr. Awótáyọ̀'s remarks, revealed that duty pervades healers' lives:

> Mo wà ní àrọ́wọ́tọ́ ní gbogbo wákàtí tí ó wà nínú ọjọ́. Kò sí ìgbà tí àwon abewé tí ó wà ní ilé ìwòsàn mi kò lè pè mí fún ìrànlọ́wọ́. Mo wà ní ibí ní gbogbo ìgbà láti ṣe ìrànlọ́wọ́ fún wọn. Nítorí náà ni mo ṣe kọ́ ilé mi sí iwájú ilé ìwòsàn mi.

> I am on call for my clients twenty four hours a day. There is no time that clients need my services that I do not respond. I am here to assist them when they need me. This is why I live right here in front of my hospital.

Additionally, I asked healers to briefly explain their experiences as a well-known traditional healer (diviner or herbalist), state how many individuals knew them in their line of work and describe how far their fame extended. I observed through the certificates and plaques hung on each healer's clinic and hospital that profiled Yorùbá Traditional Healers are prominent members of the Nigerian Traditional Healers Association, the Nigerian Native Doctors Association, *Ọ̀yọ́*, *Ògùn*, *Ọ̀ṣun*, and *Ondó* Native and Traditional Healers Associations and Association of *Ifá* Priests. I also observed that the props, cues, and artifacts displayed by the healers in their homes, clinics and hospitals show their allegiance to their professions and mentors.

The seven *babaláwo* profiled served as chairmen of their local Traditional Healers Association, including Dr Akinolá, who was the chairman of a local chapter of the Native Traditional Healers Association in *Ìbàdàn*, *Ọ̀yọ́* State in 1994. Furthermore, clients, community members, Deans of healers and elders informed me, at separate times during my field research, that all the seven Yorùbá Traditional Healers were well-known and respected in their towns, cities, states and other parts of Nigeria.

Lastly, I observed a prop with leopard skin hanging on the back of the main door at the entrance of Dr. Akinọlá's *Ọ̀yọ́* State office and saw the picture of a famous, *Yorùbá* religious leader, the late Rev. Ayọ̀ Babalọlá, in the corner of Dr. Awótáyọ̀'s office. Relatedly, Dr. Awótáyọ̀, the first Yorùbá Traditional Healer interviewed for this study, stated the following: "I admire Rev. Babalọlá, one of my mentors, because he designates Almighty God (*Olódùmarè*) as the source of his power." In the following paragraphs, I provide detailed information on the healers' and diviners' unique backgrounds and experiences.

Herbalist/*Onísẹ̀gùn* 1

Dr. E. B. Awótáyọ̀ of Awótáyọ̀ Memorial Hospital, *Ẹrìn Ìjẹ̀ṣà*, *Ọṣun* State, was 73 years old in 1994, and has been actively involved in healing mental illness for over 47 years. Like many of the healers profiled in this study, he does not have any formal Western education. When asked how he obtained the power and authority to start his healing practice, Dr. Awótáyọ̀ responded that "I inherited the power to heal psychiatric problems and illness from Akinláyẹmi, my grandfather, a healer of national and international repute, who specialized in healing "*àrùn ọpọlọ*" (brain disorders).

Dr. Awótáyọ̀ was not an apprentice to any traditional healer. Instead, he inherited the power to heal mental illness from his grandfather through observations and natural endowments. He further affirmed "the power of healing mental illness, hunting, blacksmith, and farming, runs in my blood because it is hereditary." Dr. Awótáyọ̀ clarified the above statements by noting that he enhanced his inherited healing power through observations, fasting, and incessant prayers to "*Olódùmarè*" (God Almighty). He further expounded upon these remarks in the following manner:

> Bàbá bàbá mi fi tàdúrà tàdúrà fi agbára àti ìsèwòsàn àárùn ọpọlọ fún mi nípa fífi ọwọ́ kọ mi ní ọrùn àti nípa fífi àyè fún mi láti fi ọwọ́ kọ wọn lọ́rùn padà.
>
> My grandfather prayerfully passed on the power to heal psychiatric illness to me by wrapping his arms around my neck and allowing me to reciprocate the same gesture to him.

Dr. Awótáyọ̀ explained that the interlocking and "twisting of arms" signified constancy and continuation of healing power within their family clan.

Dr. Awótáyọ̀ was chosen to be a traditional healer in his father's house, despite the fact that he was not the first son. He was selected because his grandfather's extended observations revealed that he possessed the following attributes: mercy (*àánú*), perseverance (*ìforítì)*, humility (*ìwà tútù*), love (*ìfẹ́*), and patience (*ìpamọ́ra*). These traits allowed him to become more knowledgeable concerning how his father and grandfather dispensed herbs and catered to clients' needs.

Dr. Awótáyọ̀ asserted that he had trained one of his children to be a traditional healer, while one of his nephews was undergoing training in 1994. Moreover, I observed three of Dr. Awótáyọ̀'s teenage sons actively participating with him in healing, and the dispensing of herbs and medication around the hospital. Dr. Awótáyọ̀ intended to continue a keen observation of his children's personality traits in order to train those suitable amongst them for the traditional healing profession. Consequently, he explained that it would be dangerous to pass the banner of healing to just one of these children, because of the sensitivity of the healing profession, and the danger of losing years of healing knowledge should something suddenly happen to that child. The quote summarized below further support this position.

> Iṣẹ́ yìí ti wúwo jù pé kí a gbé e lé eni tí ó láhun, tí kò ní ìgbàgbọ́, tí kò lááánú lójú, tí ó ṣánjú, tí kò ní ẹ̀mí mímọ́.
>
> This work is too delicate to be passed on to any child, especially to one who is miserly, who has no faith, is not compassionate, is callous, and who does not have the Holy Spirit.

When asked regarding Dr Awótáyọ̀'s behavior and attitude toward his clients, he informed me that "perseverance (*ìforítì*), endurance (*ìpamọ́ra*), empathy (*ìfi ara ẹni sí ipò ẹnìkejì*) and persistence (*ìdúró ṣinṣin*) in whatever I do has made my healing practice and interaction with clients successful." He reiterated his previous point by declaring that he typically overcame obstacles through constant prayers, fasting, and by utilizing the experience that he had learned in healing for his clients' advantage.

Concerning the breadth of his experience as a reputable traditional healer, Dr. Awótáyọ̀ stated that he could "capably say (makes a gesture by hitting his chest with his right palm three times to portray confidence) that I have been endowed by God Almighty to heal various types of mental illness." This confidence stems from the fact that he has over 47 years of traditional healing experience with mentally-challenged clients. Dr. Awótáyọ̀, who again made a gesture by hitting his chest with the palm of his right hand four times, claimed that he possessed the ability to successfully treat different types of mental illness when placed alongside Western-trained psychiatrists.

In support of the aforementioned point, Dr. Awótáyọ̀ noted that Professor R. O. A. Mákànjúọlá, then head of Psychiatric Unit at the Ọbáfẹ́mi Awólọ́wọ University (OAU) Teaching Hospitals Complex, and some other

Western-trained psychiatrists from OAU's Faculty of Health Sciences and elsewhere in Nigeria, routinely consult with and invite him to their departments to give lectures, and assist medical and pharmacy students.

Finally, Dr. Awótáyọ̀ averred that he offered counseling services to clients and their family members. He described himself as a traditional healer who healed mental health problems, and a counselor, father, consultant, and speaker, in addition to being a farmer who owned over 300 acres of farmland where cocoa, palm produce, herbs and vegetables are grown and maintained with the help of his wives, children and hired laborers. I observed Dr. Awótáyọ̀ dispensing *asofẹ́yẹjẹ*, one of the active herbs he grew and prepared as medication for 400 clients in his hospital, to one of his clients.

Herbalist/*Onísẹ̀gùn* 2

Dr. S. Babalọlá Akínọlá of Afrik Naturalist Hospital *Ìbàdàn*, *Ọ̀yọ́* State was 62 years old when he was interviewed in 1994. He has been involved in herbalism and general traditional healing for over 30 years. Dr. Akínọlá was a Chartered Accountant licensed in various Nigerian and International Accounting Organizations before he became a full time traditional healer, after his friends convinced him to extend his healing assistance to outsiders. Dr. Akínọlá was born into traditional healing profession, as his father and grandfather were both renowned herbalists and traditional healers. Therefore, he inherited traditional healing and knowledge of "herb mixing" from his father.

Also, Dr. Akínọlá's father taught him how to "heal and discern", beginning in 1945 when he was 10 years old. During this time, he watched and consulted with his father, and gained training in herb use, preparation and administration. Collegial relationship and respect developed between Dr. Akínọlá and his father, as a result of positive healing interactions that the respondent had with clients.

Dr. Akínọlá was licensed to practice traditional healing, which he inherited, by the Nigerian Association of African Medicine after undertaking periods of internship with different Deans of healers and experienced herbalists. He underwent special training on preservation and refinery of herbs and plants as a way of honing his hereditary knowledge of healing and herbs, under specific Deans of healers in different parts of *Yorùbá* land. In addition, Dr. Akínọlá improved his knowledge of traditional healing and "herb mixing," by undergoing a five-year apprenticeship in London under Mr. A. J. Kareem, a world-renowned traditional healer.

As a result of this specialized training, Dr. Akínọlá successfully made an effective blood tonic that was completely sold out to pilgrims during his pilgrimage to Mecca in 1968. Dr. Akínọlá, when giving me a tour of his pharmacy, said that he administered all his herbal concoctions to friends and family members before prescribing them to clients to ensure they are safe and effective. Dr. Akínọlá further explained that he was interested in dispensing medications that will be effective for his clients' ailments.

When asked whether he performed other duties/work in addition to divining/healing, Dr. Akínọlá responded in the following manner:

> Iṣẹ́ mi ni láti máa ṣe ìwòsàn oríṣiríṣi àìsàn, láti máa ta egbògi àti láti máa ran àwọn abewé àti ìdílé wọn lọ́wọ́.
>
> My work is to practice general traditional healing, dispense and sell locally—prepared herbs and medicine, and counsel individuals and their families.

Also, Dr. Akínọlá declared that he prepared and refined herbs (and medicaments) for diseases like high blood pressure, hypertension, diabetes, piles, heart conditions, stroke, and different forms of cancer. A tour of his pharmacy revealed where he stored various herbs specifically labeled for the above ailments and diseases. Most of these herbs were grown near his home and clinic in Ìbàdàn.

As evidenced by this intensive training and expertise, Dr. Akínọlá had in-depth knowledge of plants and botany. The videotaped sessions of Dr. Akínọlá's clinic showed his library, which contained various reference materials on plants, human physiology, biology, chest and heart diseases. He used these books to keep abreast of trends and modern approaches to herbs, plants, and diseases affecting all areas of the body. I observed various types of herbs as we both toured Dr. Akínọlá's herbal farm, which was adjacent to his house and hospital.

Regarding the extent of his experience as a well-known traditional healer, Dr. Akínọlá stated that he worked hard to mix and preserve herbs, and assisted clients by administering herbs that will protect them against evil forces and diseases. As such, he helped his clients to become prosperous in their business ventures, and attain long life by giving them herbs prepared specifically for these two purposes. I observed that one of the mottos (*àmì òye*) on Dr. Akínọlá's table, which supports his interest in herbs, read, "Herb Cures, Herb Heals" (*ewébẹ̀ n wòsàn, ewébẹ̀ nmú-lára-dá*).

Dr. Akínọlá has acted as a consultant to different universities in Nigeria and written on different aspects of healing for two Nigerian newspapers, *The Nigerian Tribune* and *The Daily Sketch*. He has also recorded and sold audio cassettes on traditional healing to other healers and clients.

Herbalist/*Onísẹ̀gùn* 3

Chief Jacob Abíọ́lá, of Abíọ́lá Native Hospital, was approximately 84 years old when this study was conducted in 1994. Since there was no formal means of keeping birth records in the town of *Ayégúnlẹ̀ Èkìtì* (*Ondó*

State) when he was born, Chief Abíọ̀lá was unable to accurately recall his date of birth. Nonetheless, he was able to recall the events that happened around the day he was born and guess his age based on these recollections.

Chief Abíọ̀lá has practiced traditional healing for more than 52 years and is self-taught; he does not have any formal Western education. Chief Abíọ̀lá retired from his clerical position at John Holt Limited in *Lagos* and *Ìbàdàn,* and relocated to his hometown of *Ayégúnlẹ̀-Èkìtì* many years ago to become a full-time healer, because he wanted to utilize his talents and endowments to assist clients. Like Dr. Akínọlá and before his retirement, Chief Abíọ̀lá had extended healing assistance to friends, co-workers, and relatives before becoming a full-time healer.

Chief Abíọ̀lá practiced general medicine and was also an expert in the following areas: obstetrics and gynecology, anesthetics, mental illness, general diseases and ailments; in individual, marital, infertility and family counseling. He also acted as a consultant to younger healers and Western medical experts. Chief Abíọ̀lá's position as a chief and elder in *Ayégúnlẹ̀ Èkìtì* community allowed him to counsel Chiefs, Kings, and other people of high repute.

Chief Abíọ̀lá learned the power to heal and counsel through an intensive 18-year apprenticeship and training under his maternal uncle, and through observations and dreams. His maternal uncle, Apàjẹ́polóògùn, told him when he was a young boy that he was endowed with healing attributes. Apàjẹ́polóògùn also predicted to Chief Abíọ̀lá's mother that he was going to be a renowned Yorùbá Traditional Healer.

Moreover, Chief Abíọ̀lá claimed that he augmented his healing power by being constantly self-taught through dreams. In addition to being self-taught through dreams, he learned divining methods as an intern from Pa Àjàyí of *Ìyagbà* near *Ìkọ̀lé Èkìtì* in *Ondó* State. Chief Abíọ̀lá also consulted with renowned Yorùbá Traditional Healers and diviners to enable his clients to get the best results. In the 1990s and possibly beyond, Chief Abíọ̀lá was widely known for his healing prowess in *Ondó, Ọ̀yọ́, Ògùn, Kwara, Lagos*, other *Yorùbá* States and throughout Nigeria, by Kings, Chiefs, and highly placed personalities.

Chief Abíọ̀lá, like Dr. Awótáyọ̀, was also a farmer of high repute in his community. He also specialized in career counseling using divining methods and prepared herbs for clients. He observed clients and consulted *Ifá* about their innate resources, talents and knowledge of numbers. This consultation allowed him to give clients appropriate advice on career choices. Chief Abíọ̀lá specifically remarked that he "gives this advice to my clients after observing their abilities and capabilities in different areas of learning through interactions with them and from results revealed to me by Ọ̀rúnmìlà through divining."

Lastly, the Chief stated that he was teaching one of his children, who was in high school in the mid 1990s, the fundamentals of traditional healing. Only one of his older children 'Túndé, who resided in *Adó Èkìtì*, regularly consulted with him on healing-related problems since he graduated as a traditional healer from his hospital.

Herbalist/*Oníṣ̀ẹgùn* 4

Dr. Michael Adéoyè Adésànyà, the owner of Àláfìà Táyọ Herbal Home, was born at *Òkè Àgbò* in *Ìjẹ̀bú Igbó*, in *Ògùn* State on December 4, 1912. He was the sixth out of his father's eighteen children and has practiced traditional healing for over 68 years. My videotaped recording captured the name of his Pharmacy as *Àláfíà Táyo* ("Sound Health Breeds Happiness") Medicine Store. Dr. Adésànyà reportedly acquired his power to heal and identify suitable herbs for healing different ailments from God Almighty (*Olódùmarè*), through heredity from his father, and through natural endowments.

His father was a renowned traditional healer who encouraged him to learn to mix herbs:

> Mo fẹ́ràn láti máa wòye bí a ti n po egbògi nígbà tí mo wà ní ọmọdé, mo bẹ̀rẹ̀ síí ran bàbá mi lọ́wọ́ láti po egbògi àti láti wá egbògi àti ewé tí ó lè wo oríṣiríṣi àìsan sàn láti ìgbà tí mo ti wà ní ọmọ ọdún mẹ́tàdínlógún.
>
> I loved to observe, practice with, and mix herbs when I was young, I started helping my father to prepare herbs and look for appropriate herbs suitable for curing different diseases when I was 17 years old.

In 1929 and under his father's tutelage Dr. Adésànyà successfully mixed and sold his first herbs. Until his father's death, he served as his consultant and made decisions on the choice of the right herbs for curing clients.

Like Dr. Akínọlá's, Dr. Adésànyà's father taught him how to heal and allowed him to solve difficult client problems that he found impossible to solve because they both had a collegial relationship. Dr. Adésànyà was able to undertake these tasks because he was skilled in the preparation and administration of herbs and tonics, which refine, replenish and increase blood volume. Dr. Adésànyà confirmed during videotaped recording sessions that he made some of these herbs and blood tonics from mango leaves and "*ọ̀pọ̀lọ́*" leaves.

I observed from the plaque displaying Dr. Adésànyà's degree that he had an equivalent of a bachelor's degree. Dr. Adésànyà further informed me that he was experienced in botany, biology and zoology, possessed "healing potential" and an aptitude for choosing the right herbs. Like that found in Chief Abíọ́lá's hospital, one of the plaques hanging in Dr. Adésànyà's clinic revealed an herbalist's certificate, which demonstrated his deep knowledge of anatomy and physiology. I observed and was given a tour of Dr. Adésànyà's personal library, which is stocked with the encyclopedias of medicine, anatomy and physiology, books on health and blood pathology, and personal records of herbs and plants. Finally, Dr. Adésànyà alleged that he had successfully used these records and books to cure various diseases, and to assist clients in need of psychological, psychiatric and medical healing over the last 68 years.

Dr. Adésànyà's 68-year practice had normally entailed general traditional medicine, consultations with Deans of healers and younger healers, and dispensing and selling traditionally-made medicine and blood tonic in *Ìjẹ̀bú Igbó*, *Ògùn* State. He had treated different kinds of illnesses and diseases, including blood-borne diseases with multifarious herbs, provided individual, adolescent, marital, family, fertility and infertility counseling to clients, and managed a farm.

Concerning his reputation as a healer, Dr. Adésànyà was a member of the *Ìjẹ̀bú* area, *Ògùn* State-based *Beje* Medical Herbalists Society and *Ajébámitálẹ̀* Herbalist Association, and the Chairman of the *Ìjẹ̀bú Igbó* Chapter of the Native Doctors' Association. As an elder in the community, he was well known and sought after for advice, consultation, and constant help for different individual and community problems in *Ìjẹ̀bú Igbó* town.

Although none of Dr. Adésànyà's children showed interest in becoming a traditional healer in the 1990s, one of his grandchildren ("the son of his first son") had shown some interest in learning healing methods, and herb preparation and administration:

> Ó bà mí nínú jẹ́ púpọ̀ láti má rí ọ̀kankan nínú àwọn ọmọ mi tí yóò kọ́ iṣẹ́ iṣègùn yìí, nítorí ọkàn mi n fẹ́ láti fi òye egbògi àti iṣègùn sílẹ̀ fún àwọn ọmọ mi gẹ́gẹ́ bí bàbá mi ti ṣe fún mi.
>
> I am saddened by my children's lack of interest in learning the healing job, because I want to pass the banner of healing and dispensing herbs to my children as my father did to me.

Dr. Adésànyà reiterated, squeezing his brow in sadness, that he believed that the talent and art of healing and dispensing herbs was so precious that it should not be lost with him but passed on to the next generation.

SUMMARY

The previous summaries were derived from the responses provided by Drs. Awótáyọ̀, Akínọlá and Adésànyà, and Chief Abíọ́lá to questions in the Interview Schedules. These questions are subsumed under the following five headings in Appendices B & C: "Birth," "Work Setting," "Personality," "Experience in the World," and "Interaction with Clients." In addition, the aforementioned descriptions, which are based on my personal observations, videotaped sessions, and the field notes of my personal interactions with elders, Deans of healers and with clients, reveal that Yorùbá Traditional Healers are regarded as custodians of knowledge and wisdom, and that they serve as role models in their different communities. In conclusion, the summaries presented on preceding pages indicate that Yorùbá Traditional Healers, comprising of herbalists (*Oníṣẹ̀gùn*) and diviners (*Ifá* priests), utilize their innate resources, divergent experiences, reservoirs of knowledge and expertise to aid their clients. Following the same format employed above, I discuss diviners' activities in the next section.

DIVINERS (*Ifá* PRIESTS)

Suggestions offered by the Deans of healers and my consultants encouraged me to interview the most experienced and knowledgeable diviners, priests and traditional healers in Yorùbá land for this study. The three diviners (*Ifá* Priests) interviewed, observed and videotaped for this study included Chiefs Awóyẹmí Awóreni (the *Àràbà*), Abíọ́dún Awójọbí (the *Aféódigba*), and Ọmọ́paríọlá Ọlájídé (the *Olórí Awo*). They resided in *Ilé-Ifẹ̀, Ọṣun State* (a city referred to as the cradle of the *Yorùbá*) and were 62, 72, and 73 years old respectively when this research was undertaken in 1994.

According to five clients who were present during the videotaped sessions, these three diviners were consulted for different diseases and psychological problems. For their part, the diviners explained that they acted as consultants to herbalists and other diviners in *Yorùbá* land, Nigeria, Africa and other parts of the world. Three *Ilé-Ifẹ̀*-based Deans of healers and two elders added that these three diviners (*Ifá* Priests), Chiefs *Àràbà*, *Aféódigba*, and *Olórí* Awo of *Ilé-Ifẹ̀,* are King *Olúbùṣe*, the *Ọ̀ni* of *Ifẹ̀*'s (a renowned King in *Yorùbá*land) major diviners and priests responsible for making sacrifices for *Ilé-Ifẹ̀'s* and for consulting *Ifá* oracle about the problems of the King and of all *Yorùbá*. I was informed by elders, Deans of healers, and other Yorùbá Traditional Healers that diviners (*Ifá* Priests) are well known for handling cases and problems that are linked to supernatural causation. In the next section, I present detailed information concerning the Chief Diviner's background and divining experience.

The Chief Diviner (the Chief *Ifá* Priest)

The Chief Diviner, Chief Awóreni, was the only diviner I interviewed for this study because of time constraints and the possibility of duplicating diviners' lifestyles, roles, functions and techniques. Nevertheless, I was able to understand the techniques and methods of divining through observations, interactions and by videotaping group divining activities of the three diviners' interactions with their clients.

When asked about his date of birth and upbringing, Chief Ọládélé Awóyẹmí Awóreni made the statement quoted below:

> Ọmọ ọgọ́ta ọdún lé méjì ni mí, a bí mi ní Òkè Itase ní Ilé-Ifẹ̀ ní ìpínlẹ̀ Ọ̀ṣun ní orílẹ̀ èdè Nijeria ní ọdún 1935. Mo dàgbà ní Òkè Ifẹ̀wàrà ní Ilé-Ifẹ̀ lọ́dọ̀ àwọn ará ilé ìyá mi.
>
> I am 62 years old, I was born in *Òkè Itase*, *Ilé-Ifẹ̀*, *Ọ̀ṣun* State, Nigeria in 1935, and I grew up at *Òkè Ifẹ̀wàrà* with my maternal uncle and family.

During videotaped sessions, Chief Awóreni affirmed that he was the *Àràbà* of *Ilé-Ifẹ̀* and the *Oníṣèsìn Àgbáyé*, the highest *Ifá* high priest in the world. His paternal grandfather, a renowned diviner and a prominent *Ilé-Ifè* chief who had many apprenticed diviners, was widely known for his "power to resurrect the dead ("*agbára láti jí òkú dìde*")."

Before becoming a diviner, Chief Awóreni learned mechanical engineering in *Òṣogbo, Ọ̀ṣun* State. He never went to a Western-oriented school because his father died in 1938, when he was only three years old. Although he had a personal love for divining, the Chief Diviner was reluctant to become the *Àràbà* and the Chief High Priest of the world (*Oníṣèsìn Àgbáyé*) when he was chosen because he felt inadequate to assume such a big responsibility since he lacked formal and long-term training in divining. Notwithstanding this reticence, one of *Ọ̀ọ̀ni Olúbùṣe's* Chiefs informed me that Chief Awóreni (*the Àràbà*) was widely known as a successful diviner throughout Nigeria, other parts of Africa, Cuba, Brazil and the United States of America.

As revealed by the following statement, Chief Awóreni inherited his power from a divine authority:

> Èmi ni ẹni tí Ifá mú láti jẹ oyè ilé bàbá mi, láti jẹ oyè oníṣèsìn àgbáyé, àlùfáà àti Àràbà àgbáyé ní Ọdún 1972, àti láti máa ṣe iṣẹ́ bàbá bàbá mi lọ lẹ́yìn ìgbà tí mo ti Òṣogbo dè.
>
> I was especially chosen by *Ifá* to be ordained as a chief and priest in my father's house and to carry on the divining rites for my grandfather's house, after I returned from *Òṣogbo* in 1972."

Chief Awóreni apparently acquired wisdom and the art of divining through heredity, dreams, visions, interactions with experts, and with different supernatural beings who constantly conversed with him on the streets. He added that he was curious, had an interest in traditional things and possessed a willingness to ensure that sick people got well. One of Chief Awóreni's long-term female clients, who brought her brother in for divining when I videotaped this session, confirmed that Chief Awóreni was always willing to assist his clients by listening to them.

During interactions and videotaping sessions, Chief Awóreni averred that no Yorùbá Traditional Healer (*babaláwo*) could make divining a full-time job and support his family because of restrictions in charging fees and because clients also consulted Western-trained medical doctors, herbalists, and religious healers. Hence and in addition to being a diviner (an *Ifá* priest and *Oníṣèsìn Àgbáyé*), Chief Awóreni served as a farmer, mechanic and the director of his own sawmill.

In 1994, three of his younger children were learning how to divine. Chief Awóreni maintained that younger students learn how to divine faster than older students, because the 256 *odù* or the sacred stories of *Ifá,* which have to be memorized, communicated and interpreted to clients, is easily accessible to younger, fresher and fertile minds.

On a final note, Chief Awóreni avowed that he does not allow himself to be overcome by any problem. Therefore, even though he worked hard at divining, he allowed the "ups and downs" of life to take their normal course. In response to questions about his attitudes toward clients, Chief Awóreni listed patience (*sùúrù*), perseverance (*ìforítì*), and endurance (*ìfaradà*) as the traits that allowed him to work successfully with his clients. In a similar vein, he made the following statement:

> "Mi ò ní ẹ̀mí ìgbéraga ṣùgbọ́n, mo ní ẹ̀mí ìrẹ̀lẹ̀, mo ní èmí ìfẹ́, mo máa n gba àwọn abewé mọ́ra mo sì máa n ran àwọn abewé tí ó n wá sí ọ̀dọ̀ mi lọ́wọ́.
>
> I am neither proud nor haughty but humble, loving, and receptive to clients who come to me for help.

In closing, Chief Awóreni stated that he worked with clients to identify solutions to their problems and encourage them to offer sacrifices to the gods and their ancestors for their problems without charging an initial fee, if they genuinely have no money. Chief Awóreni buttressed his genuine concern for clients' well-being by citing the following proverb:

> Wọn kìí bá ìbànújẹ́ wọlé ọba, kí wọ́n tún bá ìbànújẹ́ jáde.
>
> Individuals never enter the King's palace with sadness and go home sad.

Hypothesis 1

Based on Yorùbá Traditional Healers' responses to questions concerning how they obtained their healing and divining power or authority, it is tenable to hypothesize that Yorùbá Traditional Healers' skills, expertise, knowledge and power are learned through apprenticeship with Deans of healers, Chief diviners, and healers' fathers; through observations; natural endowment; self-teaching; genetic dispositions; or dreams; and/or close meetings and associations with God Almighty (*Olódùmarè*), the gods, ancestors and supernatural beings.

Group Divining

Professor Akin Mákindé, my chief consultant and expert on Yorùbá Traditional Healers, reiterated that the use of a three-team group divining approach with clients engenders positive outcomes. I observed that the three diviners not only worked as a team, they were cordial, cooperative, hard working, and worked collaboratively to understand clients' problems and seek divine guidance from *Ọ̀rúnmìlà* for solutions to such issues. One of the diviners informed me that "my professional interactions and cooperation enabled clients to develop confidence in my divining ability to solve most of their problems through client-healer relationships."

Yorùbá Traditional Healers' Client-Healer Relationships

Dr. Awótáyọ̀

Dr. Awótáyọ̀ affirmed that he empathized with his clients, encouraged them to take care of their personal hygiene and eat well-balanced diets, consisting of vegetables and black-eyed beans, and desired that they got well. Dr. Awótáyọ̀ also expressed love and mercy toward clients and their family members who visited his hospital. In relation, he maintained that "not being puffy (*fífẹ̀*) or full of self (*ní ìgbéraga*), and being humble (*ní ẹ̀mí ìrẹ̀lẹ̀*) allowed him to build his traditional healing profession up to its present stage." Dr. Awótáyọ̀ summed his response by informing me that healing is a work of grace and alluding to the following proverb: "*Asá kòkó pẹ̀lú kòkó rẹ̀ ni yóò gbẹ*" (The person that is drying cocoa beans in the sun will dry out just like the beans).

In order to ensure that his clients' health improved, Dr. Awótáyọ̀ provided them with the necessary assistance one hour at a time, listened to their problems, ensured that they took their medications, and helped them with healing-related issues as they arose. Moreover, he made the remarks quoted below.

> Mo máa n gbìyànjú láti ran àwọn abewé láti ṣiṣẹ́ lórí àti ní ẹ̀mí ìfaradà, ìgbàgbọ́ nínú Olódùmarè wípé oògùn tí a ó fún wọn yóò ṣiṣẹ́ tí a fẹ́ kí ó ṣe. Mo sì tún n ran àwọn abewè lọ́wọ́ nípa jíjẹ́ kí wọ́n mọ̀ pé mo máa dúró tì wọ́n títí di ìgbà tí ara wọ́n yóò yá.
>
> I encourage my clients to have patience, perseverance, endurance, persistence, faith in God Almighty that the medication that they are given will work towards their healing. I also assist my clients by making them aware that I will follow through the process of healing with them.

Dr. Awótáyọ̀ is renowned for a high success rate with his clients if they consistently took their medication for two full years (*ọdún méjì gbáko*):

> Ọ̀gọ̀rọ̀ àwọn tí ó ti ti ilé ìwòsàn wa yìí kúrò ni ó ti padà sí ẹnu iṣẹ́ wọn, wọ́n sì ti bẹ̀rẹ̀ síí ṣe ojúṣe wọn ní áàrín ìlú láì sí wàhálà kankan mọ́.
>
> Some of the clients who have been discharged from this hospital have returned to their careers and professions and become functional members of the society.

He cited numerous clients who had advanced professionally and otherwise in the community after coming for treatment in his hospital, and claimed that these examples showed how successful his hospital had been in enabling clients to get well. One of the interns at Dr. Awótáyọ̀'s hospital informed me that several clients, who left the hospital when he was a patient there, returned to show appreciation to Dr. Awótáyọ̀ now that they were working as highly placed government officials in Federal and State Ministries. According to Dr. Awótáyọ̀, none of his clients had died since he started healing over 47 years ago because they were always given special care and attention.

I observed that some of Dr. Awótáyọ̀'s old clients who had previously been in treatment at his hospital stayed behind as his students or worked in the hospital as interns. These old clients pointed out to me that they remained to assist Dr. Awótáyọ̀ because they had no relatives to pay their hospital bills when they were sick. These clients further explained that they would leave after they graduated as healers or had worked for enough years to pay their debts. A discussion of Dr. Akínọlá's client-healer relationship is the focus of the next section.

Dr. Akínọlá

One of the clients interviewed for this study declared that Dr. Akínọlá was very talented at discerning what was wrong with clients before being told about their problems. The client added that Dr. Akínọlá was endowed with the gifts of healing and problem discernment, as well as with talents to resolve different crises. For his part, Dr. Akínọlá asserted that, because he worked hard to find the root causes of and solutions to clients' problems, his over 30-year experience of traditional healing practice was characterized by multiple success stories.

Dr. Akínọlá did not treat psychiatric problems because they were time-consuming. Consequently, he conducted research, prayed, and asked questions concerning other difficult but non-mental health issues. Also, Dr. Akínọlá echoed the voices of the other Yorùbá Traditional Healers examined in this study when he made the following remark:

> Ṣíṣe áànú, ṣíṣe iṣẹ kára, ìforítì, ìrẹ̀lẹ̀, ọ̀wọ̀, níní ọkàn ìbéèrè, fífi ara ẹni sí ipò ẹnìkejì, ìfẹ́, ìbẹ̀rù Olódùmarè, ìgbàgbọ́, òye, gbígba àdúrà láìsinmi sí

Ọlọ́run jẹ́ ìpìlẹ̀ ìwà tí ó n ran babaláwo lọ́wọ́ láti lè kó esẹ̀ járí pẹ̀lú àwọn abewé.

Mercy, hard work, perseverance, humbleness, respect, a probing mind, empathy, love, fear of God, faith, understanding and constant prayer to God are the foundations of a healer's success when working with clients.

Hence, from Akínọlá's vantage point, mercy (*àánú*) is the basic foundation of Yorùbá Traditional Healing: "any traditional healer who is not endowed with mercy (*àánú*) cannot be successful in the healing trade."

Dr. Akínọlá interacted actively with his clients, and utilized his skills and expertise to solve their problems. While interacting with his clients, he employed a direct approach, which includes the use of patience (*sùúrù*), endurance (*ìforítì*), empathy (*fífi ara ẹni sí ipò ẹnìkejì*), mercy (*àánú*), love (*ìfẹ́*), probing spirit (*ẹ̀mí ìbéèrè*), discerning mind (*níní ẹmí àkíyèsí*), and maturity (*níní ẹmí àgbà).*

My observations of Dr. Akínọlá's interactions with his clients during videotaped sessions showed him asking questions about their backgrounds, work settings, eating and sleeping habits. As further evidenced through the videotaped sessions, my observations and interactions with Dr. Akínọlá and the other three herbalists, I discovered that Dr. Akínọlá's style of interaction was similar to that of Messrs. Awótáyọ̀, Adésànyà and Abíọ́lá, because they all asked relevant questions, probed the causes of clients' problems, empathized with, listened to and assisted clients to work through and find solutions to their problems.

All the profiled babaláwo averred that they were eager to help, showed mercy (*àánú*) and respect (ọ̀wọ̀), worked hard to ensure that clients' problems were solved, ensured that clients learnt the necessary preventive healing methods, showed empathy (*fi ara wa sí ipò ẹnìkejì*) and understanding (*òye*) during client-healer interactions. Finally, Dr. Akínọlá's response summed up Yorùbá Traditional Healers' unanimous belief on the issue of obtaining payment for healing:

A kìí kọkọ bèèrè owọ́ ni ọwọ́ àwọn abewé. A ó kọ́kọ́ wádìí ohun tí wọ́n bá wá, a ó sì gbìyànjú láti ràn wọ́n lọ́wọ́ nípa wàhálà kí wàhálà tàbí ìṣòro kí a tó bèèrè owó lọ́wọ́ wọn.

We do not ask for money from clients when they first visit us. We ask them to describe their problems and we try our best to help them find the solutions before asking them for money,

The next section discusses Chief Abíọ́lá's healing relationship with his clients.

Chief Abíọlá

Chief Abíọlá claimed that he utilized the healing power given to him by God Almighty to aid, rather than to hurt, his clients. His reported aim was to ensure that clients got better and were healed by responding to their needs through listening and daily interactions:

> Ọ̀pọ àwọn abewé tí ó n wá sí ọ̀dọ̀ mi ni ó n gba ìwòsàn tí wọ́n sì tún n sọ fún àwọn ẹlòmíràn nípa iṣẹ́ ribiribi tí mo n ṣe.
>
> Most of the clients who come to me not only get healed, but they also refer other clients to me for the good work I do.

Chief Abíọlá offered advice and used past experiences, including clients' success stories, to offer encouragement and suggestions as he worked through different issues with them. In a similar fashion, he made the following point:

> Ìwà rere ni ohun tí mo fi ṣe pàtàkì lẹ́nu iṣẹ mi yìí.
>
> Character is the foundation of my success in traditional healing job.

Hence, Chief Abíọlá believed that character is the crown of success. He added that since character (*ìwà*) is the cornerstone of living, if a traditional healer has character he or she will be able to interact with, and relate to others and therefore be successful in all his or her endeavors. The warm reception, which he gave his clients, encouraged them to work on their problems. This warmth is shown through the exchange of greetings and pleasantries, and expressions of goodwill between Chief Abíọlá and his clients. Overall, Chief Abíọlá mentioned that he cared for (*ṣe aájọ̀*), showed mercy to (*fi àánú hàn*), and gave full attention to the clients who came through his doors.

One of Chief Abíọlá's clients reiterated that "the chief allowed his clients to feel at home in his clinic by using appropriate words that denoted empathy (*fífi ara ẹni sí ipò ẹnìkejì*), mercy (*àánú)* and cordiality (*níní ìfẹ́*)." Relatedly, Chief Abíọlá referred to the cordial reception that he gave my entourage as an example of the way he treated his clients and their family members. Another client, who was part of the videotaped session in Chief Abíọlá's hospital, stated that he showed kindness, love, patience, and genuine love to him, his family members and other clients. In sum, Chief Abíọlá referred to genuine love and mercy as the foundation of his success in working with clients.

On a separate issue, Chief Abíọlá cited the example of a woman who was over nine months pregnant and had multiple pregnancy complications.

Although she visited Western-trained doctors in *Àkúré*, *Adó Èkìtì*, and *Ìdó Èkìtì's* major hospitals, they were unable to resolve her problems. However, using his knowledge of anatomy and physiology, Chief Abíọ́lá safely delivered the baby by employing an open attitude, divining and use incantation to cast out the spells that were responsible for blocking the baby's way, and finally applying some medication to relieve the client of any after-birth problems. This success story encouraged Western trained medical doctors from all parts of Nigeria to refer more obstetrical problems and complications, which they could not handle, to Chief Abíọ́lá.

Chief Abíọ́lá's consultation with other healers and elders all over Nigeria on healing methods, techniques, and different client problems allowed him to solve difficult problems like the one described above. Chief Abíọ́lá's pride in his work ensured that clients were treated in a respectful manner; in turn, they recommended him to their friends. Likewise, Chief Abíọ́lá treated his clients like royalty whenever they brought their problems to him individually or when accompanied by their relatives. He also added that

> Mo máa n sa ipá mi láti ran àwọn abewé tí ó n wá sí ọ̀dọ̀ mi lọ́wọ́ nípa fífún wọn ní oògùn tí yóò wo àìsàn wọn sàn. Mo sì tún máa n fetí sí ìṣòro tí wọn bá wá sí ọ̀dọ̀ mi kí n lè gbà wọ̀n ní ìyànjú léyìn ìgbà tí mo bá ti ṣe àwárí ìdí ìsòro náà pẹ̀lú wọn.

> I strive very hard to assist clients who come to seek help from me by prescribing the right herbs that will cure their illness or disease. I also listen to their problems that they bring to me to find the root causes of these problems.

Dr. Adésànyà

According to Dr. Adésànyà, his experience with clients revealed that honesty is the best policy. Consequently, he constantly encouraged his clients to be careful about revealing innermost secrets of their hearts to other human beings because he believed that trust should be earned. Hence, information about clients and self should be guarded and revealed with caution to other professionals only after they have demonstrated their ability to keep such information confidential.

Dr. Adésànyà stated that his motto of *"ìwà ló jù."* (character is the ultimate crown of success) prevailed in his relationship with clients and other individuals. Dr. Adésànyà emphasized that character (*"ìwà rere"*) was the basic foundation of his interaction with clients. In order for clients to appreciate his personal worth as a healer, he routinely advised his clients to visit Western-trained doctors before consulting him. One of Dr. Adésànyà's clients explained:

Àmọ̀ràn tí Dókítà Adésànyà gbà wá láti kọkọ lọ bẹ̀ àwọn oníṣègùn míràn wò kí a tó wá sí ọdọ wọn, fún mi ní ààyè láti mọ iyì iṣẹ wọn pẹ̀lú mi.

Dr. Adésànyà's advice that we should first visit other health practitioners before consulting him for healing, allowed me to appreciate his unique and valuable service.

In closing, Dr. Adésànyà stated that

Mo mọ̀ wịpé ọ̀gọ̀rọ̀ ẹni tí ó bá wá bá mi fún ìrànlọ́wọ́ ni ó máa rí àànú gbà, tí wọ́n sì máa lọ sí ilé wọn pẹ̀lú ayọ̀.

I know that most of the clients who visit me for help will find solutions to their problems, and go back home satisfied.

Diviner-Client Healing Relationships

The videotaped sessions and my observations of the relaxed atmosphere in which the three diviners worked with one another, support the contention that their mode of interaction is conditioned by a team approach that this group atmosphere brings to healing. I observed that the three profiled diviners worked together as a team to help clients. Chief Awóreni informed me that we chose one another as diviners because we complement each other, have similar knowledge, are all helpful to clients, possess wisdom, have similar backgrounds and experiences as Chiefs and *Ifá* priests, and are proficient in *Ifá* language. In support of Akiwowo's (1979) observation regarding the oral tradition's principle of listening and understanding communicated thoughts, the diviners added that they utilized uttered statements with varied words *(gbólóhùn)* in their conversations with their clients.

Also, the three diviners concurred that they divined individually with clients who approached them when other diviners in the team were unavailable. In reviewing the videotaped sessions, I was impressed with the way the three diviners, Chiefs Awóreni, Awójọbí, and Ọlájídé, worked together amicably through positive group interactions to solve their clients' problems. They worked corporately with a male client with marital problems who came to them at the recommendation of his sister. The clients, who were videotaped as they consulted the herbalists and diviners for treatment, felt welcomed and accepted by Yorùbá Traditional Healers in general and these three diviners (*Ifá* priests) in particular.

Diagnoses in Yorùbá Traditional Healing

I observed that the three diviners diagnosed the aforementioned client's problems by throwing their divining chain (*ọ̀pẹ̀lẹ̀*) on the mat. After some incantations, Chief Awóreni informed me, during videotaped sessions, that *Ọ̀rúnmìlà* revealed that his marital problems would be solved if the client utilized patience, wisdom, love, and made sacrifices. I listened as the chief diviner's advice was repeated by the other two diviners after throwing their divining chains on the mat. Subsequently, the client told me that he would heed the diviners' suggestions in order to have a peaceful marriage. The three diviners re-emphasized that they consulted the *Ifá* oracle using a team approach and consulted other healers when necessary to help unravel the nature of their clients' difficulties.

Customarily, Chief Awóreni inquired about the nature of clients' problems from *Ọ̀rúnmìlà*, the father of all truth and the custodian of all the hidden secrets of the universe. I observed as Chiefs Awóreni, Awójọbí and Ọlájídé allowed several clients to whisper their problems, needs or requests into Naira (Nigerian currency) notes before putting the money into a divining tray. The videotaped sessions showed the diviners throwing the *ọ̀pẹ̀lẹ̀* (divining chain) on the tray to inquire from *Ọrúnmìlà*, through the *Ifá* oracle, what clients' needs, requests, or problems were. I also observed the diviners as they explained how the *Ifá* oracle unraveled the problem(s) that the clients whispered to the divining chain (*Ọpẹ̀lẹ̀*). One of the clients informed me that the diviners' explanations of his problem(s), as revealed through the *Ifá* oracle, were completely accurate.

I observed in reviewing videotaped sessions that diviners used their innate and acquired resources to access secrets through the use of the divining chain. I also observed and listened as the three diviners repeated the same problems and solutions for one of their clients by throwing the divining chain (*ọ̀pẹ̀lẹ̀*) on the mat, interpreting and communicating the meanings revealed through *Ọ̀rúnmìlà* or *Ifá*. Moreover, I observed as Professor Akin Mákindè, the researcher's chief consultant, secretly spoke into the divining chain (*ọ̀pẹ̀lẹ̀*) about a very important issue of his life. Professor Mákindé later told me that he agreed with the diviners' interpretations and suggestions regarding the solution of the problem at hand and the revelations that came out of his whispering silently to the divining chain *("sísọ̀rọ̀ wúyẹ́wúyẹ́ sí ọ̀pẹ̀lẹ̀")*.

Two observed diviners' clients remarked that they had the option of either whispering directly to the divining chain or to the money, which was usually a N50 note or a larger denomination, whenever they visited the diviners. These two clients further declared that, before there was a deterioration in Nigeria's economy, they used to whisper into coins and not Naira bills.

According to Chief Awóreni, the last stage of diagnosis and consultation with the diviners (*Ifá* Priests) entailed a confirmation by the client that the facts *Ọ̀rúnmìlà* revealed through the *Ifá* oracle were accurate. *Yorùbá* consult and have faith in traditional healers (*babaláwo*) because revelation from *Ọrúnmìlà* supports the truth elicited through divining. One of the clients declared after his sessions with the three diviners that "*Yorùbá* clients believe that anyone who can reveal clients' innermost secrets with honesty and without probing openly, but by throwing the divining chain (ọ̀pẹ̀lẹ̀), is worthy of respect."

All the profiled Yorùbá Traditional Healers affirmed that they employed different methods to diagnose their clients' problems. Specifically, when asked to describe their modes of inquiries, Drs. Akínọlá and Adésànyà stated that they used the psycho-social-cultural-physical-social-spiritual-family model, which involved asking questions about clients' psychological, social, cultural, physiological and social interactions, spiritual stances, and families of origin, in order to garner detailed information concerning their conditions. One interviewed client remarked that Dr. Akínọlá allowed her to give as much information as possible about herself during healing interactions. Another client added that Dr. Akínọlá posed questions that covered demographical issues, psychosocial matters, work settings, eating and sleeping patterns, and the duration of existing problems.

My observations and the videotaped sessions also revealed that the four herbalists inquired about their clients' backgrounds, sleeping patterns, eating habits, work settings, and disease histories. In particular, these videotaped sessions depicted Dr. Adésànyà asking questions about dream patterns, parenting styles, discipline, parental involvement with children, especially adolescents, and the backgrounds of the "presenting problems." He also posed open-ended questions that not only helped him discover the causes of the problems, but also allowed clients to think and become involved in the healing process.

Before beginning the healing process, Dr. Awótáyọ̀ asserted that he consulted diviners, other traditional healers, and God Almighty (*Olódùmarè*) about the cause of each client's mental illness. One of his clients professed that Dr. Awótáyọ̀ fasted with his clients for many days in order to get God Almighty (*Olódùmarè*) to reveal their problem(s) and solutions to him. The videotaped sessions depicted Dr. Awótáyọ̀ observing a client's eating habits and physical fitness, and inquiring about his family background and financial status, before he was admitted to the hospital.

Through the videotaped sessions and my observations, I discovered that, before healing could occur, Chief Abíọ́lá made sacrifices after consulting diviners and other healers. He and Dr. Awótáyọ̀ agreed that it was better to consult diviners and other healers on clients' problems at the initial stage, than to wait until healing commenced to get all the facts about the illness or problem. Chief Abíọ́lá cited the example of the previously-described case of the female client with birth complications as a reason why diagnosis cannot always be done effectively by one traditional healer. He was able to deliver his client's baby after the due date, because he consulted with different diviners and herbalists who offered feedback and other assistance that allowed him to get to the root of the problem ("*wá òfin tótó ìdí àìsàn náà*").

Generally, interviewed Yorùbá Traditional Healers emphasized that they prayed to God Almighty (*Olódùmarè*), their main source of discernment, for solutions to their clients' problems. Three interviewed clients also claimed that they believed that God Almighty (*Olódùmarè*) empowered Yorùbá Traditional Healers (*babaláwo*) to cure, heal and give clients the motivation to change.

In Dr. Akínọlá's view, his success in healing stems from his endowment with the ability to identify and discern clients' problems, and identify the proper herbs for cure. Healing tools used by Yorùbá Traditional Healers to find solutions to clients' difficulties are as follows: problem identification, diagnosis, discernment, divining, seeking solutions to problems from *Orúnmìlà*, inquiring from *Olódùmarè* about the sources of clients' problems, the prescribed solutions and the appropriate herbs to be used to heal, as well as entreating or invoking the gods or ancestors where called for, and consulting other healers.

In Chapter Five, I continue with a discussion of several important themes, including healers' interventions, interactions, underlying principles of healing, techniques, treatment strategies, culture and healing, general observations, precautions and key hypotheses derived from this primary study of traditional healers.

CHAPTER FIVE

Case Facts and Hypotheses (Continued)

INTERVENTIONS IN YORÙBÁ TRADITIONAL HEALING

Chiefs Awóreni, Abíọ̀lá and Drs. Adésànyà, Akinọlá and Awótáyọ̀ employed different approaches to solve their clients' problems. A former client and an intern in Dr. Awótáyọ̀'s hospital in 1994 opined that *Yorùbá* clients often view their problems as spiritual, psychological, or physical in nature. According to Drs. Awótáyọ̀, Akinọlá and Adésànyà, the previous observation about the potential causes of a problem necessitates that Yorùbá Traditional Healers confront clients' problems from different angles every time. As such and in Dr Awótáyọ̀'s view, "a disease, illness or problem can only be solved when 'dug out from its roots' (*"wo àrùn tegbò tegbò, wo àrùn láwòtán"*)."

Chiefs Abíọ̀lá and Awóreni, and Drs. Adésànyà, Akinọlá and Awótáyọ̀ believed that they will not be regarded as successful traditional healers if their clients returned to them for treatment for the same illness, disease, or problem. Therefore, Chief Awóreni made the statement quoted below.

> Àdúrà babaláwo tí abewé kannáà bá wá n bá fún oríṣi àìsàn kannáà léèmejì kò tîì gbà ni.
>
> If a client comes back to a traditional healer with the same disease, illness or problem twice, the healer's prayers have not been answered by God Almighty.

In a similar vein, one of Dr. Adésànyà's clients attested that,

> Àwọn babaláwo fi àwa abewé sókàn wípé wọ́n gbọ́dọ̀ ràn wá lọ́wọ́ láti yanjú wàhálà, wá òfin tótó ìṣòro tàbí àìsàn tí a bá gbé wá fún wọn nípa

> lílò gbogbo agbára tí Olódùmarè fún wọn láti ràn wá lọ́wọ́ yálà nípa fífún wa ní egbògi ni, àkànṣe oúnjẹ ni, gbígbà wá sínú ilé ìwòsàn wọn ni, ṣíṣe ètùtù ni, tàbí nípa gbígbà wá ní ìyànjú.
>
> Yorùbá Traditional Healers help solve our problems by utilizing all available resources given to them by God Almighty as herbs, food, using sacrifices, invoking and entreating the gods, or admitting us into their hospitals or giving us suggestions.

Drs. Akinọlá, Awótáyọ̀, and Adésànyà and Chiefs Abíọ́lá and Awóreni contended that problems evolve to be solved in the here and now, and are not meant to be dragged on forever. I discovered through videotaped sessions and interactions with the seven Yorùbá Traditional Healers that their willingness to help clients "find meaning in the face of personal crises leads to the discovery of proactive pathways of healing" (Levers, 1996).

Furthermore, Drs. Akinọlá, Adésànyà, and Awótáyọ̀, and Chiefs Abíọ́lá and Awóreni listed knowledge of their clients and their problems, likes and dislikes, culture, family of origin, ability to be physically present with their clients and their families, as variables that help Yorùbá Traditional Healers establish trust in their dealings with their clients.

HYPOTHESIS 2

Based on responses obtained from healers and the issues highlighted in the preceding section, it is tenable to hypothesize that Yorùbá Traditional Healers concentrate on clients' physical, mental, emotional, and spiritual well-being during counseling and healing sessions.

Encounters in Yorùbá Traditional Healing

Drs. Awótáyọ̀, Akinọlá and Adésànyà, and Chiefs Abíọ́lá and Awóreni regard *Yorùbá* culture as the foundation upon which they base their merciful mode of interaction with clients. According to Chiefs Awóreni and Abíọ́lá, Yorùbá Traditional Healers' interactions depend on their areas of specialization, levels of expertise, ages, lengths of years in healing, degree of supernatural power, extent of natural endowments which aid in problem discernment, the type of problem, past success rates with that particular type of problem, knowledge of the problem, their clients and families. From Chief Awóreni's vantage point, the *Yorùbá* highly exalt any individual who can assist others with their wisdom, natural endowments, and supernatural power. Hence, he surmised that this was one of the reasons why *babaláwo* have to attain a certain minimum age (usually over 40 years old) before they can become a renowned traditional healer.

In support of the above postulation, Drs. Akinọlá and Adésànyà contended that Yorùbá Traditional Healers (*babaláwo)* must have a higher status in the community than others and be a role model, a seer, a custodian of knowledge, respectable, respectful and caring according to the rules established by Nigerian Traditional Healers, Ifá priests and State-based Healing Associations.

On their respective attitudes toward current and prospective clients, Drs. Awótáyọ̀ and Adésànyà alleged that Yorùbá Traditional Healers relate to their clients as a father figure and use appropriate *Yorùbá* healing words. They further affirmed that, in order to become effective healers, *babaláwo* must cultivate and improve their divine gifts through training, internship, consultation and supervision.

I observed through interactions with Drs. Awótáyọ̀, Akinọlá and Adésànyà, and Chiefs Abíọ́lá, Awóreni (the *Àràbà*), Awójọbí, and Ọlájídé that they served as elders within their respective communities. In 1994, Chief Abíọ́lá of *Ondó* State was a third-in-rank chief to the king of *Ayégúnlẹ̀ Èkìtì*, *Ondó* State, while Dr. Akinọlá was an Elder in *Ológèdè* Village, *Ìbàdàn*, *Ọyọ* State. Chiefs and the Kings of *Ẹrìn Ìjẹ̀ṣà*, *Ọṣun* State, and other adjoining communities, also sought Dr. Awótáyọ̀ for his wisdom and advice. When this study was undertaken in the 1990s, Dr. Adésànyà was a prominent man sought after by young traditional healers in *Ìjẹ̀bú-Igbó, Ògùn* State.

I discovered through the videotaped sessions and plaques hung in their offices, clinics and hospitals that the profiled Yorùbá Traditional Healers were also leaders within the professional body of Nigerian Traditional Healers. The Dean of healers, other Ifá Priests, chiefs and elders in *Ilé-Ifẹ̀* community informed me that Chief Awóreni was the world's greatest priest (*Oníṣèsìn Àgbáyé*) and diviner. In this position, he performed healing activities for clients and acted as a consultant to other healers in the city, in Nigeria and other parts of the world. Chief Awóreni, the chief diviner, declared that Chiefs Awójọbí and Ọlájídé were two of King Síjúadé, the *Ọ̀ọ̀ni's* (the ruler of the city of *Ilé-Ifẹ̀ and* one of the most respected kings in *Yorùbá* land and Nigeria) prominent chiefs, diviners (*Ifá* priests) and healing consultants.

Several people, including many clients I interviewed, expressed respect and awe for Yorùbá Traditional Healers' (*babaláwo's*) power, and sought them for their wisdom, knowledge and supernatural endowments. Conversely, Yorùbá Traditional Healers respected their clients, kept their problems confidential, showed them love, cared for them, and were always receptive and open to them, regardless of the problem or illness that they presented to them. By and large, Chiefs Awóreni and Abíọ́lá concluded that healer-client interactions have endured over the years because Yorùbá Traditional Healers have used their knowledge, supernatural power, appropriate communication patterns, interpretations and principles to alleviate clients' problems.

Underlying Principles of Yorùbá Traditional Healing

Yorùbá Traditional Healers create a climate of trust, acceptance, and respect for their clients. Chief Awóreni buttressed the above point by adding that,

> Mi ò lè sùn sórí ibùsùn mi kí n má dá ọkùnrin tàbí obìnrin tí ó bá wá bèèrè nípa wàhálà ayé wọn lọ́wọ́ mi lóhùn nítorí pé mi ò mọ bí nkan tí wọ́n bá wá sí ọ̀dọ̀ mi ti le tó. Mo gbọ́dọ̀ dá gbogbo ẹni tí ó bá wá bá mi lóhùn. Mi ò gbọdọ̀ gbéraga rárá nítorí mi ò gbọdọ̀ fi agbára tí Olódùmarè fún mi wọ́lẹ̀. Kí Olódùmarè má gbé ẹ̀wù ìgbéraga wọ̀ mí o, Àmín.
>
> I cannot sleep on my bed when my clients need my attention to assist them to solve their problems. I should not be vainglorious because I do not want to allow my God-given talent to be wasted. May God never allow me to be proud. May God never allow me to be cloaked with pride. Amen.

Equally, Drs. Awótáyọ̀, Akinọlá and Adésànyà, and Chiefs Abíọ́lá and Awóreni stated that Yorùbá Traditional Healers show empathy (*ìfi ara ẹni sí ipò ẹnìkejì*), mercy (*àánú*), respect (*ọ̀wọ̀*), friendliness (*fífẹ́ràn*), love (*ìfẹ́*), and create a climate of trust (*ìgbẹ́kẹ̀lé*), which they all viewed as traits necessary for engendering wholeness amongst their clients. I observed that these basic qualities helped Yorùbá Traditional Healers as they utilized different techniques with their clients.

Techniques used by Yorùbá Traditional Healers

Chiefs Awóreni and Abíọ́lá and Drs. Adésànyà, Akinọlá and Awótáyọ̀ submitted that divining, sacrifices, herbal therapies, therapeutic dances, prayers, entreating and invoking the gods and ancestors, incisions, dream interpretations, proverbs, folk tales and stories were the most common techniques used by Yorùbá Traditional Healers to solve clients' problems. I highlight these techniques in the subsequent paragraphs.

Divining

Chiefs Awóreni, Awójọbí and Ọlájídé described divining as counting, throwing and using divining chains (*ikin* or *ọpọ́n Ifá*) to inquire from *Ọ̀rúnmìlà*. Chief Awóreni specifically noted that throwing the divining chain (*ọ̀pẹ̀lẹ̀*) on a mat allows healers to inquire into clients' problems by asking *Ọ̀rúnmìlà* (the father of all gods), the question for which an answer is sought.

The Process of *Ifá* divination

According to Chief Awóreni, the chief diviner and *Ifá* priest, *Ifá* priests address several issues, including whether or not a client should embark upon a journey and important matters of life and death involving a sick person. In order to ensure that divination was successful, diviners use citation of memorized *Ifá* names or praises to Ọrúnmìlà. Chief Awóreni also declared that interpretations of the content of clients' difficulties are done by the priest or diviner. Relatedly, Epega & Neimark (1995) explained that "by casting the divining chain (*ọ̀pẹ̀lẹ̀*), the diviner (*babaláwo*) can, in a single toss, arrive at the necessary eight symbols to form a complete odù, with a seed that fall with the concave or inner surface face up equalling a single mark (I), while one that falls with the convex or outer surface face up equals a double mark (II)" (p.xv).

Chiefs Awóreni, Awójọbí and Ọlájídé attested that the first two parts of *Ifá* divination are done in a monologue as incantations by the diviners, while the last part is done with the client's participation. An incantation usually involves the uttering of words according to a formula, in a set order, to achieve a set purpose. Additionally, Chief Awóreni further explained that incantations are recited in different forms to serve the purpose of medication. I observed from the videotaped sessions that diviners threw the divining chain (*ọ̀pẹ̀lẹ̀*) on a mat to ask *Ọ̀rúnmìlà* about the nature of clients' problems during the first part of the healing process, and disclosed the interpretation revealed by *Ọ̀rúnmìlà* to the clients during the second part.

Sacrifices

Chiefs Abíọ̀lá and Awóreni and Drs. Awótáyọ̀, Adésànyà and Akinọlá stated that sacrifices (*rírú ẹbọ*), considered to be at the core of healing, empower them to solve clients' problems. One of Chief Awóreni's clients added that the ability to "follow through" with making sacrifices as the healer suggests, determined his ability to attain sound health. The videotaped sessions revealed that Chiefs Awóreni, Awójọbí, Abíọ̀lá and Drs. Awótáyọ̀ and Akinọlá, and some of their clients, listed animals and items like chickens (*adìyẹ*), goats (*ewúrẹ*), cows (*mààlúù*), snails (*ìgbín*), kola nuts (*obì*), palm oil (*epo pupa*), water (*omi*), and money (*owó*) as some of the animals and objects that are used for sacrifices.

Drs. Awótáyọ̀, Akinọlá, and Adésànyà and Chiefs Awóreni and Abíọ̀lá disclosed that making sacrifices is the first step in diagnosing client's problems. They also divulged that in certain cases, sacrifices are first performed before proceeding to ascertain the sources of clients' problems. Chiefs Awóreni and Abíọ̀lá, and Dr. Awótáyọ̀ emphasized that sacrifices could be done in healers' compounds, clients' homes, outside the city limits near a river or forest, or on a mountain.

In Chief Awóreni's view, the type of sacrifice, where it is to be done, how it is to be done, for and by whom it is done, depend on the gravity of clients' situations. Problems or illnesses that involve life and death demand prompt sacrifices that need to be performed with the help of the *babaláwo* that diagnose the problem. One of Chief Akinọlá's clients proclaimed that she promptly followed Yorùbá Traditional Healers' instructions because they are the supernatural mediators between human beings and their ancestors.

Herbarium—Herbal Therapy

The four herbalists, Drs. Akinọlá, Awótáyọ̀ and Adésànyà, and Chief Abíọ́lá, claimed that they were knowledgeable in herbal therapy, and utilized herbs and different plants to cure different ailments. According to Dr. Akinọlá, he used almond leaves on his farm for refining blood and curing blood-borne diseases. Drs. Adésànyà and Akinọlá allowed me to peruse records of all the herbs that they used to cure different diseases and ailments. They also continued to refine, experiment, test, and conduct research to discover better methods of administering herbs to their clients.

To improve their knowledge of medicinal plants and herbs, Drs. Akinọlá and Adésànyà consulted health encyclopedias and other sources for information on health, plants, botany and blood-borne diseases. I discovered through observations and interactions with Drs. Awótáyọ̀, Akinọlá and Chief Abíọ́lá that they had farms where they grew and tended herbs and plants used for medicinal purposes. Several clients informed me that they had repeatedly consulted Drs. Awótáyọ̀, Akinọlá, Adésànyà and Chief Abíọ́lá for different problems and ailments because they possessed innate and acquired knowledge of appropriate herbs that cured different mental illness, physical and gynecological conditions. One client, who was an intern within Dr. Awótáyọ̀'s hospital, was undergoing training on how to identify, mix and use herbs to improve his knowledge of healing.

Therapeutic Dances

Chief Awóreni defined therapeutic dance as the dance that enables clients to work through and gain independence from problem-related stressors. Music is an important part of daily living among *Yorùbá* and Africans. Music and dancing are used on different occasions to spur child birth, religious observations, marriages, initiations, and funerals. The three diviners (*Ifá* priests) stated that music added grace to every merrymaking occasion among the *Yorùbá*. Music allows clients to find solutions to some problems, because music, singing, listening, and dancing are used by clients for relaxation and as a means of working on their problems.

The videotaped sessions depicted a client's sister singing, dancing, and using song interpretation as a "mode of transition," while the three diviners threw a divining chain on the mat to inquire about her brother's problems. My observations also revealed the diviners assisting the client, as the sister's singing and dancing resumed after *Ifá* revealed to the diviners that the source of her brother's problem was his relationship with his wife. I also noticed that the diviners joined the client's sister in singing a song that directly told a story similar to the client's. In so doing, the diviners expected the client to relate sympathetically to the main character in this song and story about a protagonist who forgave his first wife. Diviners chose this song to highlight a conflict resolution similar to the client's and to encourage the client to use a similar method to resolve his own issues.

Prayer

Prayer is the mainstay of Yorùbá Traditional Healer's profession. In support of this assertion, Drs. Akinọlá and Awótáyọ̀ viewed Yorùbá healing as being equally underpinned by prayer and sacrifice. Consequently, Chief Awóreni affirmed that "*Àdúrà ni ẹbọ*" (Prayer is sacrifice). During my conversations with the seven healers, they emphasized that prayer could be in the form of entreating God Almighty (*Olódùmarè*), invoking the ancestors or the gods, as each client understands them, or offering sacrifices to *Olódùmarè*, ancestors, the gods, or the elders who are wiser and can give clients needed comfort and wisdom to work through their situations.

Dr. Akinọlá supposedly prayed in his prayer-room, which is adjacent to his office, for clients, prospective clients and their family members (both before and after seeing them) five times a day because he believed that healing without prayers prevent clients' problems from being solved. Additionally, Dr. Awótáyọ̀ fasted and prayed with and for his clients to get well and go home to become functional members of the community, and one of his clients described prayer as the cornerstone of healing in Awótáyọ̀'s Hospital.

Yorùbá Traditional Healers (*babaláwo*) use prayers and sacrifice to appease *Olódùmarè,* the gods and the ancestors as a process of making healing final for their clients. They say prayers on behalf of their clients to ensure that they worked through difficult and complicated problems. For Dr. Awótáyọ̀, prayer to God Almighty (*Olódùmarè*) completed the healing process for the babaláwo and his client.

One of Dr. Adésànyà's clients concluded that saying prayers to *Olódùmarè* made it relatively easy to appease the gods. Yorùbá Traditional Healers believe that God Almighty (*Olódùmarè*), the ultimate source of answered prayers and the chief ruler of the universe, made positive things happen by answering all prayerful invocations made to *Ọ̀rúnmìlà*, all the gods and ancestors on their clients' behalf.

Entreating and Invoking the gods and ancestors

Clients are advised to entreat and invoke the gods and the ancestors when *Ọrúnmìlà* entreats them to do so through the *Ifá* oracle. The following statement, expressed by Dr. Awótáyọ̀, expounds upon the previous observation:

> Ìgbàkúgbà tí Olódùmarè tàbí àwọn alágbára tí ó ju ti ẹ̀dá lọ bá fi àṣẹ fún wa pé kí a gba àdúrà tàbí ṣe ètùtù fún àwọn abewé a ó tètè yára ṣe é fún ànfàní wọn.
>
> Whenever we are authorized by Olódùmarè, the gods or any supernatural power to make sacrifice or say prayers to entreat, appease or invoke the gods and ancestors on behalf of our clients, we immediately do so for the benefit of our clients.

Yorùbá Traditional Healers believe that some clients have problems because they refuse or forget to pay homage to their ancestors or because they disrespect *Olódùmarè*, *Ọrúnmìlà* or the gods. Respect for *Olódùmarè*, the gods, supernatural beings, and ancestors are important elements of *Yorùbá* culture.

Prayer to *Olódùmarè* takes the form of pleading or entreating. In Dr. Awótáyọ̀'s hospital, clients' family members say prayers when clients are very sick and cannot talk or say the prayers themselves. Invoking and entreating the gods and the ancestors can take the form of sprinkling palm oil, blood of a chicken, goat, or cow or going to the cemetery or burial place to say prayers or ask for certain requests from long dead ancestors. All the above rites are done with the aid, support, and advice of the *babaláwo*.

HYPOTHESIS 3

Based on clients' comments, my own observations, and videotaped sessions, it is tenable to hypothesize that Yorùbá Traditional Healers believe that prayers to God Almighty (*Olódùmarè*) complete the healing process.

Incisions

Incisions (*gbẹ́rẹ́*) are small cuts made into the skin with a lancet or any other sharp instrument. Incisions are used for clients for different purposes in *Yorùbá* land. Most commonly, they are used to prevent diseases, alleviate a swollen body that is ridden with too much water and vaccinate children. Some incisions are made on the head and other strategic parts of clients' body to prevent evil from coming to clients' lives. Dr. Awótáyọ̀ often used incisions to get rid of excess water from a client's body before treating their mental illnesses, while Dr. Akinọlá alleged that his AIDS cure, made in the form of incisions, could protect clients from the HIV virus.

Dreams and Dream Interpretations

Profiled healers, including Dr. Awótáyọ̀, perceived dreams as valuable to the *babaláwo* in the conduct of their activities. Certain Yorùbá Traditional Healers sharpen their healing knowledge and obtain instructions about how to solve difficult problems from dreams. The videotaped sessions showed that suitable herbs were revealed to Drs. Awótáyọ̀, Akinọlá, and Adésànyà, and Chiefs Abíọ́lá and Awóreni through dreams. Chief Awóreni also stated that he learned how to divine through dreams and meetings with supernatural beings.

During healing and counseling sessions, Drs. Awótáyọ̀ and Adésànyà asked their clients about their most recent dreams. One of Dr. Adésànyà's female clients informed me that she dreamt that her dead father saved her from disaster several times. She added that Dr. Adésànyà interpreted this dream to mean that her ancestor was closely watching over and protecting her. Dr. Adésànyà later made some recommendations that allowed this client to relate her dream to solutions of the problem that she brought to counseling. Dreams, according to Dr. Adésànyà, enabled *babaláwo* to learn more about their client's problems and gain insight into hidden mysteries that can only be revealed by *Olódùmarè*, *Ọ̀rúnmìlà*, the gods, and the ancestors.

Proverbs

The *Yorùbá* regard proverbs as intellectual maps that the wise use to find lost paths in the world. When asked "what other points can you add to the above that I have forgotten to ask you," Chief Awóreni replied that this question was an "*adébẹamọ̀*" (additional question that enhances knowledge). More particularly, he stated that a *Yorùbá* proverb is referred to as *òwe*: "*Òwe ni ẹṣin ọ̀rọ̀, tí ọ̀rọ̀ bá sọnù òwe ni a fií wá a*" (Proverb directs language, if a word is lost, proverbs are used to find it).

Yorùbá Traditional Healers' explanations of proverbs is supported by Adégbìtẹ́'s (1993) reference to *babaláwo's* use of language as being closely linked with the *Yorùbá* belief in the power of the spoken word. Adégbìtẹ́ (1993) added that the spoken word has some hidden symbolic and inexplicable implications or importations with its utterance producing the desired effect without the use of magical or medicinal preparations.

Yorùbá Traditional Healers use proverbs to instill wisdom into their clients. The videotaped sessions showed Dr. Adésànyà telling a wife that came for marital counseling that "*sùúrù lè se òkúta jinná*" (patience, perseverance, and endurance can cook a stone until it becomes soft and tender). Dr. Adésànyà explained the above proverb as meaning that perseverance, hard work, and endurance enable a wife to enjoy a fruitful marital life. Drs. Awótáyọ̀, Akinọlá, and Adésànyà and Chiefs Abíọ́lá and Awóreni used the proverb, "*Sùúrù ni baba ìwà*" (patience is the foundation of character), at different times during the course of my interviews.

Many of the healers constantly emphasized in their responses that,

> Iwà tí ó jẹ́ ọba àwúre ni aláşeyọrí ohun tí ó ṣe pàtàkì nígbà tí a bá n jíròrò pẹ̀lú àwọn abewé tí ó n wá sí ọ̀dọ̀ wa.
>
> Character, the crown of success, is the basis of how we interact with our clients.

Yorùbá Traditional Healers use language as the vehicle for undertaking traditional healing. They use proverbs as a successful traditional healing and counseling tool, and to instill wisdom into and get their points across to their clients.

Folk Tales and Stories

Folk tales (*ààlọ́, ìtan*) are common ways of transmitting tradition, knowledge and wisdom to others in *Yorùbá* land. Most teachers utilized folk tales to instruct their students and to pass tradition on from older to younger generations before the advent of writing. Yorùbá Traditional Healers walked clients through delicate and problematic situations by reenacting stories about what they have seen happen, or telling stories from *Ifá* oracle, from their healer fathers or mentors, or using stories to identify the actions of main characters as role models or teachers. Chief Abíọ́lá added that he learned healing by listening to stories from successful healers and through *Ifá* oracle teachings.

The videotaped sessions revealed Chief Awóreni and his team of diviners telling the story of how a brother, who forgave his brother who attempted to kill him, later became a rich and prosperous ruler. The three diviners acknowledged that this story helped instill wisdom into the life of one client who was observed for this study.

Generally, diviners use folk tales from ancient *Yorùbá* literature when revealing secrets to clients during *Ifá* divination sessions. In the same vein, Epega & Neimark (1995) stated that diviners communicate and interpret the odùs, the sacred stories of *Ifá*, which have survived through *Yorùbá* oral tradition. They further contended that "each odù carries with it hundreds of tales that have accumulated in the oral tradition of *Ifá* through thousands of years" (p. xvii).

HYPOTHESIS 4

Following from the preceding analyses, it is tenable to hypothesize that Yorùbá Traditional Healers use divining, sacrifices, herbal therapies, therapeutic dances, entreating and invoking the gods and ancestors, incisions, dreams and dream interpretations, proverbs, folk tales and stories and family-supported counseling as techniques that help clients better manage their lives.

Sources of the Techniques used by Yorùbá Traditional Healers

Most of the techniques used by Yorùbá Traditional Healers are attributed to God (*Olódùmarè*), as the *Yorùbá* believe that God is the giver of all supernatural or natural power. Interviewed healers stated that their techniques, which produce positive healer-client interactions, are given from dreams by God Almighty (*Olódùmarè*), through inherited characteristics and skills, learned from *Ọrúnmìlà* and their superiors, or as part of *Yorùbá* tradition or culture.

Yorùbá Traditional Healers' Interactional Approaches

Drs. Awótáyọ̀, Akinọlá, and Adésànyà and Chiefs Awóreni and Abíọ́lá regarded mercy *(àánú)* and character (*ìwà)* as requisite for successfully healing clients. Likewise, they maintained that the following are needed to make healing a success: Concern *(aájò*), lending a helping hand *(ìrànilọ́wọ́*), and non-pretentious love (*ìfẹ́ àìṣetán*), hard work (*iṣẹ́ àṣekára*), endurance (*ìfaradà*), perseverance (*ìdúró ṣinṣin*), patience (*fífi ara balẹ̀*), persistence (*ìtẹramọ́ṣẹ́*), keen observation (*ìkíyèsí tìtaratìtara*), humility (*ìrẹraẹnisílẹ̀*), esteeming others (*gbígbé ènìyàn lárugẹ́*), sacrificial giving (*kí ènìyàn má ṣe ahun*), listening to elderly advice (*gbígbọ́ràn sí àwọn àgbà lẹ́nu*), respectful attitude (*kíkún fún ọ̀wọ̀*) and consulting with others who know more about the profession (*fífi ọ̀rọ̀ ẹni lọ àwọn tí ó mọ̀ jù wá lọ*).

Yorùbá Traditional Healers further listed assistance *(ìrànlọ́wọ́*), encouragement (*gbígba ẹni níyànjú*), exemplary behavior *(ìwà rere tí ó ran ẹlòmíràn lọ́wọ́*), role modeling (*ìwà tí a lè lò fún àpẹrẹ*), kindness *(inú rere)*, and being there for clients (*ìnítara*) as behaviors and attitudes required to create and maintain solid healer-client relationships. In particular, they employed empathy and mercy with their clients because *babaláwo* work through problems with their clients. Several times during my interviews, Drs. Awótáyọ̀, Akinọlá and Adésànyà and Chiefs Abíọ́lá and Awóreni stated that,

> *Babaláwo* tí kò bá ní àánú kò lè kó ẹsẹ járí nínú iṣẹ́ ìwòsàn yìí.
>
> Any *babaláwo* who is not merciful cannot be successful in the healing profession.

Chief Awóreni and Dr. Awótáyọ̀ summed it up with the statement quoted below.

> Iṣẹ́ yìí ti wúwo jù pé kí a gbé e lé ẹ́ni tí kò l'áànú lójú lọwọ.
>
> The healing trade is too delicate to be passed to an individual who has no mercy (àánú).

According to Dr. Awótáyọ̀ and Chief Awóreni, individual healers who find it difficult to show mercy often misuse the power and techniques passed on to them by *Olódùmarè* to destroy rather than to aid clients. All the seven Yorùbá Traditional Healers referred to *mercy* as an important skill necessary for the success of traditional healing.

HYPOTHESIS 5

Based on the foregoing discussions, it is tenable to hypothesize that Yorùbá Traditional Healers consider mercy (*àánú*), character (*ìwà*), kindness (*inú rere*), assistance (*ìrànlọ́wọ́*), concern (*aájò*), encouragement (*gbígba'ni níyànjú*), hard work (*iṣẹ́ àṣekára*), endurance (*ìfaradà*), humility (*ìpamọra*), esteeming others (*pípọ́n èniyàn lé*) and patience (*fífi ara balè*) as requisite for inducing successful healing outcomes with their clients.

Healer-Client Healing Interactive Interrelational Strategies

Yorùbá Traditional Healers create a climate of trust, relaxation, love, acceptance, respect, atmosphere of positive acceptance, receptability, empathy, and unparalleled mercy through their interactions with clients during healing. Drs. Awótáyọ̀, Akinọlá and Adésànyà and Chiefs Abíọ́lá and Awóreni opined that a serene climate allows clients to talk and think about their problems, and start moving towards healing.

This climate of trust, peace, acceptance, love and mercy creates a positive restorative effect that commences before the healing interaction actually begins. Clients visit the *babaláwo* with faith that they will receive help. One of Dr. Awótáyọ̀'s clients explained that this positive expectation allows clients from all walks of life to come into healing interactions with the hope that everything will be all right once they see and talk with the *babaláwo*. The above client and one of Chief Awóreni's clients both admitted openly that consultation among Yorùbá Traditional Healers guarantees effective healing outcomes. Clients consult Yorùbá Traditional Healers daily on matters relating to marriage, having a baby, traveling, career choices, naming a child, starting a trade and solving marital problems because they respect, admire, trust, have faith in and adore traditional healers.

HYPOTHESIS 6

As evidenced by the previous comments, it is tenable to hypothesize that Yorùbá Traditional Healers' use of care, empathy, love, respect, compassion, patience, hard work, consistency, faith in God Almighty (*Olódùmarè*), constant prayer, a probing mind, fear of God, humility, attention to details of clients' problems, eagerness to offer services, continual presence with their clients spur positive therapeutic and healing outcomes.

YORÙBÁ TRADITIONAL HEALERS' TREATMENT STRATEGIES

Dr. Awótáyọ̀

Dr. Awótáyọ̀ remarked that his relationship with clients revealed empathy, respect, love, mercy, joy, patience, humility, and faith that they will get well. My observations and comments elicited from five interviewed clients showed that the doctor cordially interacted with and greeted his clients, and later attempted to resolve their problems. I also observed Dr. Awótáyọ̀'s full commitment to all his clients at the hospital. Clients are allowed to remain in treatment until they are well enough (*gba ìwòsàn lágbàtán*) to go home and become functional members of the society. The number of years for hospital stay is usually between one to three years for some clients, including the two years they have to come and take their medication.

Dr. Awótáyọ̀ gives his clients taboos (*èèwọ̀*) that they should refrain from both when they are in the hospital and when they leave. One of the five clients interviewed in Dr. Awótáyọ̀'s hospital, who said that he has been advised to refrain from using salt, asserted that these *taboo* (*èèwọ̀*) are usually in the form of foods like a large rat (*òkété*), salt (iyọ̀), sugar (*iyọ̀ dídùn*), rice (*ìrẹsì*), pounded yam (*iyán*), and alcoholic drinks (*ọtí líle*).

Dr. Awótáyọ̀ reported that he empathized with his clients by paying special attention to them and by treating them as unique individuals. He claimed that his special wish and prayer for clients were that God Almighty (*Olódùmarè*) should heal them and that they should go back to former or better vocations.

Dr. Awótáyọ̀ studies the underlying problems prevalent with the client and his or her family before healing the client. Close family members like mothers, fathers, sisters, cousins, aunts, nieces and nephews, take turns to observe, stay with, help administer medication, and attend family sessions during in-patient and outpatient sessions in Dr. Awótáyọ̀'s hospital, which is about 90 kilometers from Dr. Akinọlá, the second herbalist interviewed for this study.

Dr. Akinọlá

One of Dr. Akinọlá's clients informed me that she had full confidence in Dr. Akinọlá's ability to solve her marital problems. She was very confident that Dr. Akinọlá was equipped to handle any illness or problem. During one of the videotaped sessions, I observed Dr. Akinọlá working with one of his clients to solve her marital problems by suggesting that they come for family counseling. He further suggested that this couple explore all avenues for having another baby. Afterwards, Dr. Akinọlá explained to me that this couple presently had a four-year-old. The client lauded Dr. Akinọlá's empathy, love, mercy and ability to convince both her husband and herself to come for counseling and healing sessions in his office, and added that,

> Oníṣègùn Akinọlá yiò ràn wá lọwọ láti yanjú ìṣòro tí a bá wá sí ọ̀dọ̀ rẹ̀.
>
> Dr. Akinọlá will help us to solve the problems that we came to him for.

Chief Abíọ́lá

Chief Abíọ́lá depicted character (*ìwà*) as the secret key behind his success with clients and of utmost importance in any healing relationship. He submitted that, if a *babaláwo* possessed character, he will be successful in all his healing endeavors. During the course of my conversations with him, Chief Abíọ́lá cited caring (*ṣíṣe aájò*), assisting others (*ríran'ni lọwọ*), empathy (*fífi ara ẹni ṣí ipò ẹnìkejì*), hard work (*ṣíṣe iṣẹ kára*), endurance (*ìfaradà*), perseverance (*ìforítì*), being considerate (*gbígba ti ẹlòmíràn rò*), and being observant (*níní ẹ̀mí ìwòye*) as traits necessary for effective healing.

Chief Abíọ́lá emphasized that being respectful ("*bíbọ̀wọ̀ fún*"), being inquisitive ("*títọsẹ̀ lọ́fintótó*"), giving others preference over myself ("*pípọ́n ènìyàn lé*'), humility ("*ìwà ìrẹ̀lẹ̀*"), kindness ("*ìṣoore*"), receptivity to others ("*fífa ènìyàn mọ́ra*), giving older and experienced women preferential respect so that they can share their expertise and knowledge with him ("*gbígbé àwọn obìnrin àgbàlagbà ní arugẹ kí wọn lè ràn mí lọwọ*"), giving his time, talents and abilities to aid clients without complaining ("*sísa gbogbo ipá mi láti ran àwọn abewé tí ó n wá sí ọ́dọ́ mi lọ́wọ́ láì ráhùn*"), as additional skills and expertise that contributed to success as he counseled and healed clients. He also attributed his accomplishments to his persistence ("*títẹramọ́sé*") and consultations with Deans of healers and *Ifá* Priests all over Nigeria ("*gbígba àmọ̀ràn lọ́dọ̀ àwọn àgbà babaláwo àti aláfọ̀ṣẹ ní gbogbo orílẹ èdè Nijeria*").

One of Chief Abíọ́lá's clients and her family declared that Chief Abíọ́lá listened, showed empathy, respect and genuine love, provided advice where necessary; dispensed herbs with utmost care, was attentive, and treated his clients' secrets with utmost confidence ("*bo àṣírí abewé*"). Finally, Chief Abíọ́lá added that he was honest with all the clients who visited him. While smiling, he admitted to me that he took special care of himself to prevent burnout and contracting other people's diseases.

Dr. Adésànyà

Equally, Dr. Adésànyà stated that having mercy (*àánú*) and specified treatment goals for each client, encouraging clients that everything will be all right, being there for clients at all times, cooperating with clients and encouraging their family members to be active in their treatment enabled him to solve clients' problems. He also proclaimed that,

> Mo ní òye àti máa ṣe aájò, àti ní ẹ̀mí ìfẹ́, fífi ara ẹni sí ipò ọmọnìkejì, ní àánú lójú, ní ẹ̀mí ìgbọ̀ràndún, ẹ̀mí ríran'ni lọ́wọ́ pẹ̀lú ẹ̀mí àgbà sí àwọn abewé tí ó n wá sí ọ̀dọ̀ mi.
>
> I exhibit the skills and characteristics of caring, love, empathy, compassion, sympathy and fatherly compassion toward my clients.

Dr. Adésànyà consulted with trusted colleagues, *Ifá* Priests and Deans of healers about his clients' progress, their family status, backgrounds, physical conditions, and psychological, social, religious, medical and emotional concerns when he treated them. According to one client, Dr. Adésànyà's caring attitude and concern encouraged him to help clients before asking them for money. Relatedly, Dr. Adésànyà said that "money cannot buy caring and compassion that we, Yorùbá Traditional Healers give," and that, after having settled down in their career and/or business endeavors, some of his clients returned to show their appreciation.

Dr. Adésànyà, like Dr. Awótáyọ̀ of *Ẹrìn Ìjẹ̀ṣà*, *Ọ̀ṣun* State, was confident that he could solve some of the problems that Western-trained medical experts, counselors, social workers, psychiatrists, and psychologists could not solve. Dr. Adésànyà's confidence derived from his knowledge of herbs, *Yorùbá* culture, human personality, clients, their families, culture, likes, dislikes, and problems. A client who traveled from *Ọ̀yọ́* to *Ògùn* State to consult with Dr. Adésànyà about his wife's barrenness, asserted that Dr. Adésànyà's physical presence promotes healing and clients' growth as individuals.

Skills needed for success in Yorùbá Traditional Healing, according to Dr. Adésànyà, included concern (*àníyàn*), love (*ìfẹ́*), compassion (*ìbákẹ́dùn*), empathy (*fífi ara ẹni sí ipò ẹnìkejì*), fatherly interaction with clients, confidence (*níní ìgbẹ́kẹ̀lé*), trustworthiness (*nìní ìgbẹ́kẹ̀lé nínú*) and wisdom (*ọgbọ́n*). In a similar vein, he made the following statement:

> Agbára láti ní ìmọ̀ nípa wàhálà tàbí ìṣòro abewé, àti láti tètè fún abewé ní ìmọ̀ràn tí ó ṣe pàtàkì nínú iṣẹ́ ìṣègùn, jẹ́ òye pàtàkì tí ó n jẹ́ kí oníṣègùn ṣe àṣeyọrí ní ilẹ̀ Yorùbá.
>
> The ability to discern, diagnose and identify problems early in the counseling sessions, offer advice and a willingness to offer precautions against future problems for clients are other skills needed to be a successful Yorùbá Traditional Healer.

Also, Dr. Adésànyà affirmed that being merciful (*lílánú, níní ìyọ́nú*), respectful (*kíkún fún ọ̀wọ̀*), having treatment goals for all clients, and keeping clients' problems and discussions confidential enabled clients to obtain healing and become whole.

Dr. Adésànyà used a direct mode of interaction when he asked pertinent questions concerning how clients' problems evolved. I discovered from a videotaped session of Dr. Adésànyà's interaction with a female client that, in helping the woman to improve her adolescent daughter's attitude, Dr. Adésànyà encouraged the woman to become positively involved in her child's life, set consequences for her negative behavior patterns, and discipline her when necessary. The sessions portrayed Dr. Adésànyà recommending that the woman return for family counseling with her daughter and husband to work on the issues of setting boundaries. Dr. Adésànyà specifically recommended a minimum of once a month family meeting after he had gained knowledge of the mode of interaction between the client and her daughter.

During Dr. Adésànyà's counseling of this female client, he recreated *Yorùbá* tradition by explaining and emphasizing parental roles vis-à-vis children's roles in the home. He did this by encouraging this mother to become a role model for her daughter, train her in character development and live an exemplary life in their home. Dr. Adésànyà related his own experience as a father to demonstrate that her client's family problems were solvable.

Diviners' Treatment Strategies

Chief Awóreni echoed the views of other interviewed *babaláwo* when he stated that Yorùbá Traditional Healers should be humble and not utilize their power to hurt or project evil intentions toward others. This remark supports Epega & Neimark's (1995) observation that *babaláwo's* successful healing method "demands humility" (p.viii).

I listened to Chief Awóreni, the Chief *Ifá* Priest, repeating the following prayer, several times with both hands clasped and raised toward the sky: "*Kí Olódùmarè má gbé ẹ̀wù ìgbéraga wọ̀ mí o*" (May God never cloak me with pride). The three diviners (*Ifá* Priests) also emphasized that a successful relationship between Yorùbá Traditional Healers and their clients is characterized by humility and wisdom. The three diviners utilized wisdom through songs, proverbs, folk-lore and witty sayings as they diagnosed and treated their clients' problems.

Treatment Strategies: Concluding Discussions

Drs. Awótáyọ̀, Akinọlá and Adésànyà and Chiefs Abíọ́lá and Awóreni reportedly accepted their clients by showing them respect, love, care, mercy, and love at all times. As a general rule, Yorùbá Traditional Healers are physically present to offer their best efforts to clients in all situations and for all problems. In their dealings with clients, Yorùbá Traditional Healers listen, attend to their needs, give advice and encouragement where necessary, give positive feedback, make suggestions, empathize, are attentive, treat clients' secrets with the utmost confidence and respect; and seek to build trust and rapport with them.

Yorùbá Traditional Healers are trusting, have an unbiased mind towards clients and their family members, and are always eager to help. In line with the dictates of the *Yorùbá* culture, where honor, prestige and status are automatically accorded to people who possess wisdom, understanding, and natural as well as supernatural power to heal and counsel, they employ direct approaches while interacting with their clients. These approaches allow Yorùbá Traditional Healers to guide, introduce information, suggestions, content, and attitudes that promote proactive and positive healing.

Yorùbá Traditional Healers also work hard to teach their clients preventive measures against diseases and problems. Healers persevere with clients by leading them toward solutions to their problems and illnesses. *Babaláwo* pray for their clients to be healed of most ailments, show humility, and work with patience, kindness, endurance, and perseverance to get to the root of their clients' difficulties. In addition, Yorùbá Traditional Healers use their cordiality as catalysts for inducing healing in their clients. Typically, *babaláwo* exhibit joy and faith in the fact that clients will get well, as they prayerfully assist them and their family members to confront their problems with optimism.

Yorùbá Traditional Healers' knowledge of herbs and various techniques engender success as they help build their clients' trust and confidence. *Babaláwo's* position within their different communities and their knowledge of *Yorùbá* culture are instrumental to the positive outcomes expected from healing and counseling sessions. Healers demonstrate their genuineness and concern with fatherly compassion as they encourage and cooperate with clients. Their ability to ask pertinent questions encourages clients and their family members to tackle their problems with ease. Yorùbá Traditional Healers take care of their clients wholeheartedly until healing occurs, until their counseling needs are met or until they can locate the source of their ailments (*wá òfintótó ìdí àìsàn náà*).

YORÙBÁ Traditonal HEALERS' UNIQUE ROLE IN THE COMMUNITY

Drs. Awótáyọ̀, Adésànyà, and Akinọlá and Chiefs Abíọ́lá and Awóreni asserted that they "stood out" as unique individuals in their respective communities and states. As noted in Chapter IV, Chief Awóreni, the *Àràbà,* is also the Chief *Ifá* Priest and diviner of the world (*Oníṣèsìn Àgbáyé*), while Chief Abíọ́lá is the *Eisikin* of *Ayégúnlẹ̀ Èkìtì,* consulted by the people of *Ayégúnlẹ̀ Èkìtì* for solutions to individual, family, community and city crises. Dr. Adésànyà was a leader within professional healing organizations, a church warden and also a community leader in *Ìjẹ̀bú Igbó, Ògùn* State. The plaques and certificates displayed in the clinic and hospitals of Drs. Awótáyọ̀ and Akinọlá showed that they were renowned members of different professional Traditional Healing Organizations.

Yorùbá Traditional Healers are keenly sought for their knowledge and wisdom by dignitaries, other traditional healers and clients within the city, the state, the country, the African continent and indeed other parts of the world. Western-trained medical doctors, psychiatrists, pharmacy professors, counselors and members of other healing-related disciplines consult *babaláwo* for their knowledge, wisdom, and understanding of herbs and healing methods. The above roles performed by healers support's the following observations made by Lámbò (1974):

> ... in addition to being a medicine man, something of a social worker and probation worker, teacher, priest, and Justice of the Peace (JP), Yorùbá Traditional Healers tackle the problem, of which his patient's symptoms are only a part, with an across the-board-approach impossible to the fragmented social, penal, and medical services in the West" (Lámbò, 1974, 33–34).

Yorùbá Traditonal Healers' Roles and Functions

To a great extent, traditional healers' roles within the *Yorùbá* community depend on people's expectations. The *Yorùbá* rely on *babaláwo* to perform different roles at different times. Chief Abíọ̀lá explained how he used water from the snail's internal organs as anesthetics for preventing bacteria from entering a male circumcised after his birth, while Dr. Awótáyọ̀ explained the process of using incisions to remove excess water from the body of one of his clients.

Yorùbá expect *babaláwo* to be there for them at all times and for different problems. Clients expect healers to address problems like infertility, child-delivery complications, marital difficulties, parental problems, mental health issues and workplace conflicts. The following comments by Dr. Adésànyà support the above observation:

> Kò sí ohun tí wọn kìí bá wá sí ọ̀dọ̀ wa, bí wọ́n ti n bá wa náà ni à n gbìyànjú láti ṣe ìrànlọ́wọ́ fún wọn nípa wọn.

> There is no problem that they do not bring to us; we put in all efforts to assist them as they bring these problems to us.

Yorùbá Traditional Healers cure a magnitude of diseases and take care of clients with multifarious concerns, and Dr. Akinọlá affirmed that Yorùbá

Traditional Healers have a type of medication referred to as "*gbogbonṣe*" (a panacea that can cure diverse ailments, diseases and illnesses). *Babaláwo* utilize their power, prestige, and knowledge to enable clients to make the best of their situations within *Yorùbá* culture.

During my field research, I observed that Yorùbá Traditional Healers assisted clients who came to them with problems ranging from career choice, handled by Chief Abíọ̀lá from *Ondó* State, juvenile delinquency, handled by Dr. Adésànyà, the traditional healer from *Ògùn* State, marital conflict, handled by Chiefs Abíọ̀lá, Awóreni, Awójọbí and Ọlájídé, and Dr. Adésànyà, and healing individuals with psychiatric disabilities, alcoholism and drug abuse as handled by Dr. Awótáyọ̀ from *Ọ̀ṣun* State.

At various times and in their daily interactions with their clients, Yorùbá Traditional Healers perform the roles of medical practitioner, psychiatrist, pharmacist, herbal dispenser, consultant, career, genetic, group, individual, marital, and family counselor, orthopedist, pediatrician, obstetrician, anesthetist, mediator, Justice of the peace, mental health practitioner, psychotherapist and crisis interventionist. Yorùbá Traditional Healers take care of their clients' physical, spiritual and psychological problems concurrently. Drs. Awótáyọ̀ and Adésànyà and Chief Abíọ̀lá addressed clients' psychiatric problems, while Dr. Awótáyọ̀ directed his own psychiatric hospital, where he acted as counselor, psychiatrist, nurse, herb dispenser, surgeon, family counselor, and pharmacist. Yorùbá Traditional Healers' ability to function as priest-physician-consultant-counselor-case worker-peace maker-mediator-pharmacist allows clients to gain holistic health, and resolve their physical, mental, psychological and spiritual problems.

Chief Awóreni's words sum up the thoughts and plans of Yorùbá Traditional Healers toward the clients who approach them for help:

> A fẹ́ ran àwọn ènìyàn tí ó bá wá sí ọ̀dọ̀ wa lọ́wọ́ tó bẹ́ẹ̀ tí ó jẹ́ wípé wọn kò ní padà wá mọ́; bíkòṣe láti dúpẹ́ tàbí láti mú ẹlòmíràn wá fún ìrànlọ́wọ́. Àdúrà babaláwo tí abewé kannáà bá n padà wá bá kò tíì gbà ni. Olódùmarè má jẹ̀ kí a ṣe àṣetì o, nítorí, àṣeyọrí ni alákàn máa n ṣe epo, àṣeyọrí ni a ó ma wo ènìyàn sàn, Àmín.
>
> We strive to help those who come to us promptly and effectively so that they do not have to come back again, except to show gratitude or bring another relative or friend for healing. The prayers of any healer, to whom the same client repeatedly comes for help for the same problem, have not been answered. May God never let us fail in all our healing endeavors because the crab never fails at making oil and may we successfully cure all who come to us, Amen.

Hence, Yorùbá Traditional Healers want their clients to be healed and assisted every time they come for help for different ailments or problems.

In explaining their quest for client healing, Dr. Awótáyọ̀ informed me that,

> A gbọ́dọ̀ tọ́jú àwọn abewé tọkàntọkàn, bí ẹni pé ìkannáà ni wá, tó bẹ̀ẹ̀ tí wọn yóò fi sàn tán pátápátá, tí wọn kò sì ní fi padà wá mọ́, ju wípé láti dúpẹ́, tàbí láti wá gba ògùn fún ọdún méjì gbáko, lẹyìn èyí tí wọn kò ní padà wá mọ́.
>
> We must take special care of our clients to ensure that they do not have to come back except to express their gratitude or get their medications for two years, after which they do not have to come back again.

In sum, Yorùbá Traditional Healers' techniques allow them to combine individual healing and counseling, where necessary, with group and family counseling and healing where applicable.

Culture and healing

Interviewed healers pointed to culture as an important foundation in healing, divining and counseling clients. Culture plays a significant role in healer-client interactions. Clients visit and feel comfortable with *Yorùbá* healers who share their worldview and speak the same language as they do. Two clients from both Drs. Adésànyà and Akinọlá's clinics explained that a comfortable, relaxed, reliable, viable, helpful, and useful healer-client relationship occurred because clients and healers are both from the same culture and operate under the same belief system. *Babaláwo* combine the roles of teacher, seer, diviner, healer, adviser, listener, and father. The fact that clients understand these roles from a cultural standpoint allows the interaction to yield fruitful results and steers the relationship towards positive results.

HYPOTHESIS 7

Following from previous analyses, it is tenable to hypothesize that effective counseling and healing occur because Yorùbá Traditional Healers share the same culture, experience, understanding, world view and view of disease, illness and problem with their clients.

Yorùbá Traditional Healers' Techniques and Cultural Norms

Yorùbá Traditional Healers and their clients clearly understand the cultural language of interaction. Relatedly, Adégbìtẹ́ (1991) explained that *babaláwo's* language is used with clients to serve "the purposes of persuasion, education, naming, greeting, entertainment, healing, conjuring and recording experiences" (p. 8). My interviews and interactions with Yorùbá

Traditional Healers suggested that the techniques of sacrifices, dreams and dream interpretations, incisions, folk tales, proverbs, prayers, herbarium, entreating and invoking the gods and ancestors, therapeutic dances, and songs are all core parts of *Yorùbá* culture.

These techniques are widely used and recognized by clients as they consult Yorùbá Traditional Healers regarding their problems. Chief Awóreni's client's sister alleged that those who recommended their friends and relatives to *babaláwo* automatically understood the healers' day-to-day routine because most of them were old clients who had successfully sought healers' help. She added that these old clients informed new clients about the process of healing and what to expect.

Usually, Yorùbá Traditional Healers are proud that their clients understand their basic approach to healing and recommend, others to visit a *babaláwo*. Clients consult healers with confidence and peace of mind because Yorùbá Traditional Healers assist their clients with their problems, utilizing the same world view, culture, religion, and a traditional base that they have grown up to understand.

HYPOTHESIS 8

Based on prior discussions, it is tenable to hypothesize that *Yorùbá* culture plays a predominant role in clients' beliefs, healers' diagnoses and the techniques of healing and curing diseases, illnesses and problems.

THE FAMILY: A CATALYST IN YORÙBÁ TRADITIONAL HEALING

The influence of the family is firmly felt in *Yorùbá* Traditional Healing, as the family is actively used as partners-in-progress for advancing clients' health and well-being. Dr. Awótáyọ̀ attested that, of the 400 clients admitted to his psychiatric hospital in 1993, only 80 clients were there without their relatives. 80 percent of his clients came to his hospital with their mothers or immediate family members. Consequently, extended family members play an active role in healing among the *Yorùbá,* as healing and questions relating to health are initiated by concerned relatives.

Family members are present through all the stages of healing to show their support, love, and caring attitude. Relatives sleep and eat with the client, when necessary, to facilitate his or her healing. In Dr. Awótáyọ̀'s hospital, the client is released early to the family member(s) when he sees involved family commitment. The *Yorùbá* believe that "*ìrọrùn ẹyẹ ni ìrọrùn eku*" (the comfort of the bird is also that of the rat); if all family members are healthy, everyone will be happy and comfortable.

The process of group healing and counseling is widely used by all Yorùbá Traditional Healers. In fact, healing is regarded as a family affair among the *Yorùbá* and families are actively involved in daily decisions pertaining to the client's life in the healer's clinic. Owing to this reality, the family emerges as the major catalyst for sound health in *Yorùbá* Traditional Healing. Dr. Awótáyọ̀ and Chief Abíọ́lá both inform the client when she or he comes in for treatment that his or her family's involvement is mandatory or recommended. The healer and his family support the client when the client's family cannot participate because of the long distance to the healers' clinic, estrangement from family members, or fear of being held responsible for relatives' hospital bills or sudden death while in the hospital. In such cases, friends, co-workers, neighbors, supervisors, and distant relatives fill the void for clients who have no relatives because *Yorùbá* believe that *ẹbí ènìyàn ni aṣọ wọn* (family members are as clothes that must be worn at all times). The belief about the importance of the family not only permeates *Yorùbá* culture, standards, and values, it successfully extends to healing practices across *Yorùbá* land.

HYPOTHESIS 9

It is tenable to hypothesize, following from previous observations, that community-oriented therapy is a culturally-appropriate and suitable method for treating *Yorùbá* clients.

General Observations of *Yorùbá* Traditional Healers

My observations indicated that Yorùbá Traditional Healers are relaxed and comfortable with their clients during healing and counseling sessions. Healers use appropriate healing and counseling techniques to address their clients' problems, who, in turn, develop confidence in the traditional healers' competence, authenticity and efficacy, because the initiative was always there to address such issues at any time of the day. In a similar vein, Chief Awóreni, the *Àràbà,* stated that,

> Ọ̀pẹlẹ mi máa n wà ní àpò mi nígbà gbogbo láti ran àwọn abewé lọ́wọ́, yálà ní ibi iṣẹ́ mi ni tàbí ní ọjà, tàbí ní àsìkò tí mo wà ní ìpàdé, nítorí a kò lè mọ irú wàhálà tí ó n pọ́n abewé lójú. Mo gbọ́dọ̀ sa gbogbo ipá mi láti ràn wọ́n lọ́wọ́.
>
> My divining beads are always in my pocket to assist clients anywhere they need my help, be it at my avocation, in the market place, or even when I am at meetings, because you never know what problems the clients may have or are working through. I must be there for them at all times.

Fees charged by Yorùbá Traditional Healers

On the above matter, Chief Awóreni made the following postulation:

Kò sí babaláwo tí ó lè fi owó tí ó pa nípa iṣẹ́ awo gun ọkọ̀ ayọ́kẹ́lẹ́

No babaláwo can ride a car from money earned solely from healing as a vocation.

The Bill of Rights of the Association of *Ifá* Priests and Yorùbá Traditional Healers' Association stipulate the fees that all Yorùbá Traditional Healers must charge. Certain profiled healers declared that any *babaláwo* who charges above the prescribed fees would never prosper. They reiterated that clients returned to express their gratitude and pay homage to healers by bringing gifts during annual festivals.

In addition to being full-time healers, Drs. Awótáyọ̀, Akinọlá and Adésànyà and Chiefs Abíọ́lá and Awóreni worked as farmers, accountants, or sawmill director to supplement their incomes. Despite their very busy schedules, the healers still found time to take care of their clients' needs.

Time and Yoruba Traditional Healers

Babaláwo take their time to cater for their clients' problems, demands, needs and problems. They are skillful, efficient, capable, always on time and attuned to their clients' concerns. *Yorùbá* Traditional Healers' skills and confidence, coupled with their ability to ensure that clients' predicaments are promptly resolved, allow them to help as many clients as possible.

Diviners usually spend more time with their clients than herbalists. Diviners (*Ifá* Priests) use a team approach that promotes effectiveness, thoroughness, and the ability to locate the root of the problem by inquiring from *Ọ̀rúnmìlà*, through *Ifá* divination, into the source of client's problem(s). The duration of time spent with each client and her or his family depends on the nature of the problem. I observed that diviners spent one hour and thirty minutes with a male client and his family member in order to assess and analyze his problem, and recommend appropriate solutions.

In explaining the process of *Ifá* divination Epega & Neimark (1995) concluded that "the *babaláwo* uses his skills to interpret the *odù* as it applies to the specific situation and presents his client with the tales or stories that express that specificity; . . . once the correct interpretation has been presented to the client, he/she and the *babaláwo* can explore specific solutions or alternatives" (p.x).

Yorùbá Traditional Healers do not allot specific time to their clients when they start working with them. Dr. Adésànyà's words echoed the assertions of the other healers when he said that,

Ẹ̀yin ni ẹ máa n topinpin nípa àsìkò, àwa kò bìkítà nípa àsìkò, nítorí wípé a ní àsìkò púpọ láti ṣe ìtọ́jú àwọn abẹ̀wẹ̀ tí ó n wá sí ọ̀dọ̀ wa, dídùn inú wa ni wípé kí a ràn wọ́n lọ́wọ́ láti gbádùn tán pátápátá lâì padà wá fún wàhálà kannáà, kìí ṣe láti ka oye abẹ̀wẹ̀ tí a ó rí àyè ràn lọ́wọ́ ní ọjọ kan.

Western trained professionals are the ones who worry about time; we don't. We have plenty of time to assist our clients; our ultimate goal is not how many clients we see per day, but how many of them acquire healing and do not have to come back with the same problem.

Yorùbá Traditional Healers work from dawn to dusk to assist their clients and family members. According to Dr. Awótáyọ̀, "*a sá kòkó pẹ̀lú kòkó rẹ̀ni yóò gbẹ*" (the owner of cocoa beans will become as dried out as the beans left in the sun while watching over them). Chief Abíọ́lá and other healers believed that their ability to willingly and ungrudgingly spend as much time as needed with their clients made them effective healers.

Precautions on becoming a Yorùbá Traditional Healer

Finally, like other professions, traditional healing offers some warnings that should be heeded by students, interns or new trainees. Healers, including Drs. Adésànyà and Awótáyọ̀, routinely cautioned their students not to utilize healing methods and supernatural power endowed on them to hurt their clients or people who their clients detest.

Summary

This chapter discussed the information that I gathered through Yorùbá Traditional Healers' responses to the questions in the interview schedules, client(s) feedback, observations and interactions via videotapes, participant observations and journals. Furthermore, I delineated nine hypotheses from the data collected and presented them in Chapters Four and Five. In the following chapter, I present a summary of Chapters One through Five, the hypotheses, an outline and discussion of related observations, and offer recommendations for further study.

CHAPTER SIX

Discussions, Summary, Related Observations and Recommendations

The major purpose of this volume was to critically and fully examine the roles and functions of, and behaviors exhibited by, Yorùbá Traditional Healers (*babaláwo*) of Nigeria toward their clients. Furthermore, this analysis generated hypotheses concerning the interpersonal techniques used by healers with their clients within the Yorùbá cultural milieu. Following from the foregoing, this final chapter summarizes Chapters One through Five, highlights the hypotheses formulated in Chapters Four and Five, discusses the observations and images that were captured during the videotaped sessions, presents recommendations for further study and analyzes implications for counselors.

Summary of the Chapters

Chapter One introduced the focus and subject area of this project and explained the aims of this project, which was to explain the interpersonal techniques used by Yorùbá Traditional Healers of Nigeria and thereafter generate relevant hypotheses. Cultural and methodological contexts, support for the volume's inductive hypotheses-producing method, the need for the study, important/critical concepts, names and terms, and a general overview of the study's methodology were also discussed in Chapter One.

The review of related literature was discussed in chapter Two. Due to the lack of pertinent data on interpersonal techniques used by Yorùbá Traditional Healers in particular, Chapter Two reviewed related literature on the subject of traditional healers in general. Major areas of the reviewed literature were as follows: ethnomedicine, personalistic and naturalistic etiologies, disease and illness, alternative medicine, cultural issues as it related to traditional healers, myths and superstitions, tradition, traditional systems of healing, traditional healers, roles and functions of traditional healers, herbalists' roles, religious healers, techniques used by traditional healers, props and cues, healing factors in traditional therapy, counseling and Western trained counselors, and guidance and counseling in Nigeria.

Chapter Three outlined and discussed the methods and procedures employed in undertaking the study. Specifically, it provided support for the use of the case study method in carrying out the investigation of the interpersonal techniques used by Yorùbá Traditional Healers of Nigeria. The chapter described the setting—*Ọ̀yọ́, Ògùn, Ondó* and *Ọ̀ṣun* States of Nigeria, where members of the *Yorùbá* ethnic group of Nigeria reside and provided a description of the subjects—consisting of four herbalists, Drs. Awótáyọ̀, Akínọlá, Adésànyà and Chief Abíọ́lá, and three diviners, Chiefs Awóreni, Awójọbí, and Ọlájídé.

Moreover, Chapter Three discussed the data collection procedures and methods utilized for the purposes of data analyses. The experiences of each individual healer and those of the Yorùbá Traditional Healers as a whole were analyzed through in-depth references to the physical, interpersonal and private or personal worlds (Binswanger, 1962) of each Yorùbá healer.

In Chapters Four and Five, I presented detailed case information and pertinent hypotheses. The case history information was discussed under the traditional healers' physical world, which describes where the healers live and perform their duties; interpersonal world, which describes the healers' interactional activities with their clients; and their private or personal world, which describes all pertinent information about each of the healers and their family members. The hypotheses formulated from these results are summarized in the following section.

HYPOTHESES

The hypotheses of this work were derived inductively from the facts of the case, which I collected using participant observation methods, interview schedules, semi-structured interviews, journal keeping records and video taping to assess the interpersonal techniques of Yorùbá Traditional Healers (*babaláwo*). In direct accordance with the case study method, this work formulated nine hypotheses based primarily upon the facts of the case and data gathered through the different methods mentioned earlier.

1. Yorùbá Traditional Healers' skills, expertise, knowledge and power are learned through apprenticeship with Deans of Healers, Chief Diviners, and healers' fathers; through observations; natural endowment; self-teaching; genetic dispositions; or dreams; and/or close meetings and associations with God Almighty (*Olódùmarè*), the gods, ancestors and supernatural beings.
2. Yorùbá Traditional Healers concentrate on their clients' physical, mental, emotional and spiritual well-being during counseling and healing.
3. Yorùbá Traditional Healers believe that prayers to God Almighty (*Olódùmarè*) complete the healing process.

4. Yorùbá Traditional Healers use divining, sacrifices, herbal therapies, therapeutic dances, entreating and invoking the gods and ancestors, incisions, dreams and dream interpretations, proverbs, folk tales and stories, and family-supported counseling as techniques that help clients better manage their lives.
5. Yorùbá Traditional Healers consider mercy (*àánú*), character (*ìwà*), kindness (*inú rere*), assistance (*ìrànlọ́wọ́*), concern (*aájò*), encouragement (*gbígba'ni níyànjú*), hard work (*iṣẹ àṣekára*), endurance (*ìfaradà*), humility (*ìpamọ́ra*), esteeming others (*pípọ́n ènìyàn lé*), and patience (*fífi ara balẹ̀*), to be the basic foundations for successful healing outcomes with their clients.
6. Yorùbá Traditional Healers' use of care, empathy, love, respect, compassion, patience, hard work, consistency, faith in God Almighty (*Olódùmarè*), constant prayer, a probing mind, fear of God, humility, attention to details of clients' problems, eagerness to offer services and continual presence with their clients spur positive therapeutic and healing outcomes.
7. Effective counseling and healing occur because Yorùbá Traditional Healers share the same culture, experience, understanding, world view, view of disease, illness and problem with their clients.
8. *Yorùbá* culture plays a predominant role in clients' beliefs, healers' diagnoses, and in the techniques of healing and curing diseases, illnesses and problems.
9. Community-oriented therapy is a culturally-appropriate and suitable method for treating *Yorùbá* clients.

Related Observations

Videotaped sessions of Drs. Awótáyọ̀, Akínọlá and Adésànyà and Chiefs Abíọlá and Awóreni revealed that Yorùbá Traditional Healers were cordial, and openly welcomed me. Relatedly, they gave open, honest, and authentic feedback that allowed me to gain insights into traditional healing and opened avenues for recommending areas for fruitful future research that will be helpful both now and in the coming years.

This volume examined Yorùbá Traditional Healers'(YTHs) techniques interactions and relationships with their clients. My research elicited information about what Yorùbá Traditional Healers do with their clients to effect positive outcomes. Discussions about Yorùbá Traditional Healers and clients responses indicated that clients have confidence in what healers do in *Yorùbá* land, and that clients from all walks of life consult Yorùbá Traditional Healers in large numbers. Additional support for clients' confidence is buttressed by the fact that certain Western trained professionals in *Yorùbá* land who hold Yorùbá Traditional Healers in high esteem also consult them for assistance in solving their clients' physical and psychological problems. Yorùbá Traditional Healers who make unique contributions to clients' overall health and wellness have a lot to offer *Yorùbá*, Nigerians, Africans, and the international community.

In the main, the responses of clients, Deans of healers, Chiefs and Elders revealed that Yorùbá Traditional Healers interact with clients because of familiarity with culture, language and traditional affinity, and because traditional healing occupies a central place within counseling and the broader cultural milieu. Responses from clients also showed that they believe that motivation to change is God-given. This spiritual spark results in high motivation for clients to get better because they perceive Yorùbá Traditional Healers as God Almighty's (*Olódùmarè's*) messengers and one of their main sources for acquiring healing. This religious/spiritual component that directs clients to look at their involvement with God Almighty (*Olódùmarè*), other gods, and their ancestors undergirds the interpersonal techniques used by Yorùbá Traditional Healers.

Yorùbá Traditional Healers' responses to questions in Appendices B & C of the Interview Schedule revealed that they view power to heal as emanating from a supernatural source. Healers pointed to this supernatural component as the foundation that gives *Yorùbá* clients faith to consult, and believe in the efficacy and authenticity of, traditional healing.

The results described in Chapters Four and Five also suggested that Yorùbá Traditional Healers regard clients as members of their own family and that they utilize care, empathy, mercy and respect when relating to them. Similarly, they maintained that clients' family members are perceived as integral parts of their treatment plans and goals. Yorùbá Traditional Healers also exclude financial constraints from being a precondition for treatment, and they claim that clients are neither ignored nor dismissed because they have no money.

The videotaped sessions revealed that there is a recognizable moral system in Yorùbá Traditional Healing practice that is based upon an empathetic perception of the client as just another human being like the healer. Interactions with Yorùbá Traditional Healers and their clients indicate that healers regard being cured as a total and permanent attainment of a certain level of consciousness or wellness. To Yorùbá Traditional Healers, *"ìwòsàn láwòtán" i.e.* being totally cured or healed, does not result in recidivism of the illness in the practice of *Yorùbá* healing.

Additionally, this work supports the contention that the training programs of both Western and non-Western nations must be infused with counseling methods that reflect different cultures (Saleh, 1989). Therefore, this volume highly supports Saleh's recommendations that the profession of counseling needs to discard monoculturalism, and become culturally reflective and relevant, since counselors' roles are shaped by the culture and circumstances in which they are working (Abonta, 1986).

In closing, Yorùbá Traditional Healers' activities are culturally reflective and successful because their roles are shaped by *Yorùbá* culture and by the circumstances and the environment in which they operate. Not surprisingly, Yorùbá Traditional Healers transmit the social, political, moral and educational norms of the *Yorùbá* culture. The results presented herein support Torrey's (1986) proposition that, regardless of what one believes about the desirability of promoting or not promoting the use of indigenous therapists in third world cultures, the fact remains that such therapists are today the only psychotherapeutic, available and accessible source of health care for the majority of the world's population. The fact that Yorùbá Traditional Healers are usually consulted by clients from all works of life for different illnesses, diseases and problems before their Western-trained counterparts, makes a thorough examination of their techniques all the more imperative.

Recommendations for Future Research

This section outlines the recommendations for further work on the interpersonal techniques used by Yorùbá Traditional Healers of Nigeria due to the paucity of literature in this area. The recommendations were also formulated from the insights gathered through discussions of observations, videotaped sessions, clients' feedback, Deans of healers' and Elders' feedback and Yorùbá Traditional Healers' responses to questions from the Interview Schedules in Appendices B & C.

Therefore from the above observation(s), it is recommended that:

1. Further research be conducted on traditional healers, utilizing the results of this present undertaking, on the techniques, models, and methods of counseling that are cognizant of African, Nigerian, and *Yorùbá* culture, since techniques of application in counseling are not automatically transferable from the Western to the traditionally well-developed and grounded culture (Mar'i, 1982).
2. More studies be conducted and published in *Yorùbá* land and in other parts of the world to identify traditional healers' levels of interactions and their exceptional performance with their clients.

Since the present volume has opened avenues for professionals to proceed to learn more concerning the valuable services offered by Yorùbá Traditional Healers, it is further recommended that experts:

3. Continue with research into the interpersonal techniques used by traditional healers in other parts of the world.
4. Test the nine hypotheses generated from this research on Yoruba Traditional Healers with traditional healers from other parts of the world.
5. Identify if there are parallels or differences between the skills, techniques, beliefs, basic foundations for therapeutic outcomes with clients.
6. Identify how healers from other parts of the world learn their skills and knowledge.

7. Identify how healing and counseling occur in different communities of the world.
8. Identify the role of culture in traditional healing elsewhere to perceive if there are parallels between the findings of this research on Yoruba Traditional Healers and the results derived from similar investigations in other parts of the world.

Future Research Strategies

Future research endeavors could include methods of healing, healing relationships, interactions between the traditional healer and his or her client, one herbalist and another, diviners, and herbalists (*oníṣègùn*) and diviners (*Ifá* priests). Specific research is required on the success rate and recidivism of traditional healers who specialize in treating clients with mental illness, alcohol and drug addiction.

Research into herbs that result in successful cures for deadly diseases like sickle cell anemia, Acquired Immune Deficiency Syndrome (AIDS), diabetes, high blood pressure, stroke, heart attack, and blood-borne diseases should, on the one hand, compare Nigerian and other African Traditional Healers, and experts on alternative medicine, counseling and traditional medicine, with other related but non-African professionals.

Inter and intra-disciplinary research on different cures for diseases and successful healing methods, and counseling techniques among medical experts, counselors, counselor educators, psychologists, psychiatrists, social workers, human service workers, sociologists, anthropologists, scientists, pharmacists, experts on alternative medicine and traditional healing should be encouraged. Research should also be undertaken on the importance of cultural influences of traditional healers on clients' health. The effectiveness and authenticity of Yorùbá Religious Healers, and *Yorùbá* Religious Healers' techniques and their interactions with clients, should also be investigated.

Nigerian counselors should be encouraged to further research traditional healers' models, techniques, and approaches that are rooted in *Yorùbá*, Nigerian and African culture. Research that will expand the literature on traditional healers should be promoted in Nigerian graduate psychology and counseling programs. Finally, legal and ethical issues as well as the applicability of this study's results to other contexts (to determine if there are parallels in techniques used and approaches with clients) should be explored.

Implications for Counselors

African, Nigerian and international counselors can learn from what traditional healers do by observing, questioning, interning and consulting with them, and by conducting first-hand research into their techniques and styles of interactions. Professors and students could advance their understanding of traditional healing with more research in this field through published articles, and through presentations on healers' techniques, interactions, and other strategies that have characterized Yorùbá Traditional Healers since the beginning of time.

Where Do We Go From Here?

Pursuant to the analyses thus far, the World Health Organization (WHO) should continue to explore avenues for an open forum for discussions between traditional healers and Western-trained counselors, social workers, rural and village health workers, psychologists, pharmacists, alternative medical experts, and Western-trained medical experts to find solutions to the problems of healing in all parts of the world.

The days when traditional healing is regarded as 'primitive', unrefined, and confined only to rural communities are gone. This research has demonstrated that all healers, traditional or Western-trained, in any part of the world, can learn a lot from each other, provided that they are willing to lay aside inherent biases and prejudices that are presently depriving the human population of access to holistic health. As Levers & Maki 1994) conclude in their study with healers in Lesotho, Swaziland, and Zimbabwe, the human services and rehabilitation service delivery systems must accept the array of professionals—Western trained and indigenous—providing interdisciplinary care to citizens in these and other countries.

Traditional healing should be reflected in multicultural studies' curriculum because differences in healing methods and techniques are means not an end. The end result for all healers (traditional or Western-trained) is to help clients solve their problems, which could be physical, physiological, psychological, emotional, mental, marital, family-related, gynecological, spiritual, or parenting issues.

It is hoped that this volume on interpersonal techniques used by Yorùbá Traditional Healers would pave the way and serve as the impetus for further research into the fascinating and worthwhile realm of traditional healers. The usefulness of such research will undoubtedly expand our knowledge of traditional healing and enable clients to benefit from alternative healing methods.

Summary

In total, the chapter summarized Chapters One through Five, discussed and enumerated the results of this volume by highlighting hypotheses, observations and interpretations. The chapter also discussed recommendations for further study, future research strategies, and implications for counselors and professionals in human services.

The chapter incorporated ideas discussed in earlier studies by Saleh (1989), Abonta (1986), Torrey (1986), and Mar'i (1982), and also highlighted the importance of encouraging dialogues between traditional and Western-trained practitioners under the auspices of the World Health Organization and other fora. Furthermore, Chapter Six enumerated the significance of utilizing the expertise, knowledge, and distinguished innate resources used by three diviners (*Ifá* priests) and four herbalists (*onísègùn*), the Yorùbá Traditional Healers profiled in this study.

References

Abas, M. A., Broadhead, J. C., Mbape, P., & Khumalo-Sakatukwa, G. (1994). Defeating depression in the developing world: A Zimbabwean model. One country's response to the challenge. *British Journal of Psychiatry, 164*, 293–296.

Abímbọlá, W. (1964). *Ìjìnlẹ̀ Ohùn Ẹenu Ifá*, (Vols. I & II). Glasgow: Collins.

Abímbọlá, W. (1968). *Ifá as a body of knowledge*. Lagos notes and Records (Lagos), 2(1), 30–34.

Abímbọlá, W. (1977). *Ifá divination poetry*. New York: NOK.

Achebe, C. C. (1986). *Training and certification of counselors: Problems and prospects*. Paper presented at the 10th Anniversary Convention of the Counseling Association of Nigeria (C.A.N.), August 3–6.

Ackerkrecht, E. (1943). Psychopathology, primitive medicine, and primitive culture. *Bulletin of the History of Medicine, 14*, 30–67.

Adégbìtẹ́, Wálé (1993). Somc fcaturc of language use in Yorùbá traditional medicine. *African Languages and Culture, 6* (1), 1–10.

Adégbìtẹ́, Wálé (1991). Aspects of language use in Yorùbá traditional medicine. *African Notes, 15*, (1–2), 7–19.

Adekson, M. O. (1987). Administration of guidance and counseling in Nigeria: Ọ̀yọ́ State as a case in view. Master of Education Thesis, Ọbáfẹ́mi Awólọ́wọ̀ University, Ilé-Ifẹ̀, Nigeria. *Masters Abstracts*, (1993), 1352491, 3104M, 1443.

Adekson, M. O. (1985). *The role of guidance and counseling in 6–3-3–4 Nigerian educational system*. Unpublished term paper written for "Administration of Guidance and Counseling," class at Ọbáfẹ́mi Awólọ́wọ̀ University, Ilé-Ifẹ̀.

Adémúwàgún, Z. A. (1978). Àláfíà— The Yorùbá concept of health— Implications for health education. *International Journal of Health Education, 10*, 35–37.

Africa Yearbook and Who's Who (1995). London: African Journal Limited.

Agyepong, I. A. (1992). Malaria: Ethnomedical perceptions and practice in an Adangbe farming community and implications for control. *Social Science and Medicine, 35*(2), 131–137.

Akérèle, O. (1987). The best of both worlds: Bringing traditional medicine up to date. *Social Science and Medicine, 24* (2), 177–181.

Alland, A., Jr. (1964). Native therapists and Western medical practitioners among the Abron of the Ivory Coast. *Transactions of the New York Academy of Sciences, 26*, 714–725.

Allport, G. W. (1937). *Personality*. New York: Holt and Rinehart.

Alonzo, A. A. (1984). An illness paradigm: A conceptual exploration of a situation-adaptation perspective. *Social Science and Medicine, 19(5)*, 499–510.

Ambler, M. (1994). Taking care of our own: Training Indians to heal Indians. *Tribal College, 5(3)*, 10–16.

Ary, D., Jacobs, L. C. & Razavieh, A. (1979). *Introduction to research in education.* Second edition. New York: Holt, Rinehart and Winston.

Asúni, T. (1990). Nigeria: Report on the care, treatment and rehabilitation of people with mental illness. *Psychosocial Rehabilitation Journal, 14*(1), 35–44.

Asúni, T. (1979). Modern medicine and traditional medicine. In Z. A. Adémúwàgún, J. A. A. Ayọ̀dé, I. E. Harrison, & D. M. Warren, (Eds.), *African therapeutic systems* (pp. 176–181). Waltham, Massachusetts: Crossroad Press.

Auge, M. (1989). From illness to words. *Psychiatrie Francaise, 20* (Special Issue), 9–17.

Awanbor, D. (1982). The healing process in Africa psychotherapy. *American Journal of Psychotherapy, 36*, 206–213.

Awolalu, J. Omosade (1979). *Yoruba beliefs and sacrificial rites.* London: Longman.

Barker, R. G. (1968). *Ecological psychology.* CA: Stanford University Press.

Baro, F. (1990). Rwanda: Mental care for all. *World Health*, 26–27.

Bascom, W. R. (1969). *Ifá divination: Communication between gods and men in West Africa.* Bloomington: Indiana University Press.

Bascom, W. (1969). *The Yorùbá of southwest Nigeria.* New York: Holt, Rinehart, and Winston.

Becker, H. S. (1968). Social observations and social case studies. In *International Encyclopedia of the Social Sciences (Volume 11).* New York: Crowell.

Beeson, P. & Scott, R. B. (Ed.)(1986). *The Oxford companion to medicine, vol I (A-M).* New York: Oxford University Press, 39–40, 219–223, 247, 314, & 416–421.

Binswanger, L. (1962). *Existential analysis and psychotherapy.* New York: Dutton.

Binswanger, L. (1968). *Being in the world.* New York: Basic Books.

Boas, H. M. (1964). *History of science.* Washington: Service Center for Teachers of History.

Bulus, I. (1989). Towards a traditional model for counseling care in Nigeria. *International Journal for the Advancement of Counseling, 12*, 105–112.

Cassidy, C. M. (1994). Unravelling the bell of string: Reality, paradigms, and the study of alternative medicine. *Advances, 10* (1), 5–31.

Chassam, J. (1967). *Research design in clinical psychology and psychiatry.* New York: Appleton-Century-Crofts.

Comaroff, J. (1980). Healing and the cultural order. The case of Baralong boo ratshidi of southern Africa. *American Ethnologist, 7*, 637–657.

Cone, C. A., & Pelto, P. J. (1969). *Guide to cultural anthropology* (rev. ed.). Glenview, IL: Scott, Foresman.

Cowan, L. G. (1987). Africa. In *The Encyclopedia Americana International ed., Vol. 1*, 256–260. Danbury, CT: Grolier.

Davis, P. W., Boles, J. & Tatro, C. (1984). Dramaturgy of occult practitioners in the treatment of disease and dysfunction entities. *Social Science and Medicine, 19,* (7), 691–698.

Denga, D. I. (1983). The state of counseling in Nigeria. *International Journal for the Advancement of Counseling*, 6(2), 115–123.

Dennett, R. E. (1968). *Nigerian studies*. London: Frank Cass.

A Dictionary of the Yorùbá Language (1991). Ìbàdàn: University Press Limited.

Denzin, N. K. (1970). *The research act: A theoretical introduction to sociological methods*. Chicago: Aldine Publishing Company.

Denzin, N. K. (1970). *Sociological methods: A source book*. Chicago: Aldine Publishing Company.

Diallo, Y., & Hall, M. (1989). *The healing drum: African wisdom teachings*. Rochester, VT: Destiny Books.

Dillon-Malone, C. (1988). *Mutunwa Nchimi* healers and wizardry beliefs in Zambia. *Social Science and Medicine, 26,* 1159–1172.

Dossey, L. (1994). Antonovsky's perspective may not go far enough. *Advances, 10*(3), 13–15.

Drewal, M. T. (1992). *Yoruba ritual: performers, play, agency*. Bloomington: Indiana University Press.

Dubos, R. (1959). *Mirage of health: Utopias. Progress and biological change*. New York: Anchor Books.

Easthope, G. (1986). *Healers and alternative medicine: A sociological examination*. Hants, England: Gower.

Edwards, F. S. (1983). Healing and transculturation in Xhosa Zionist practice. *Culture, Medicine, and Psychiatry*, 7, 177–198.

Edwards, S. D. (1986). Traditional and modern medicine in South Africa: A research study. *Social Science and Medicine*, 22(11), 1273–1276.

Eliade, M. (1964). *Shamanism: Archaic techniques of ecstasy*. Princeton: Bollingen Foundation.

Eliade, M. (Ed.). (1987). *The encyclopedia of religion*. New York: Macmillan.

Epega, A. & Neimark, P. J. (1995). *The sacred Ifá oracle*. San Francisco: Harper.

Eskin, M. (1989). Rural population's opinions about the causes of mental illness, modern psychiatric help sources and traditional healers in Turkey. *The International Journal of Social Psychiatry, 35*(4), 324–328.

Essen, A. J. A. (1972). Towards an indigenous philosophy for guidance in Nigeria. In M. O. A. Dúrójaiyé (Ed.), *Psychological guidance of the school child*. Ìbàdàn: Evans Brothers, 102–13.

The Europa World Year Book (1995). London, England: Europa Publications Limited.

Ezeji, P. N. & Sarvela, P.D. (1992). Health care behavior of the Ibo tribe of Nigeria. *Health Values—The Journal of Health Behavior-Education and Promotion, 16*(6), 31–35.

Fábùnmi, Chief M. A. (1975). *The efficacy of indigenous counseling*. Nigerian Careers Council. Ìbàdàn, Nigeria: University of Ìbàdàn.

Fabrega, H. Jr. (1990). Psychiatric practice and the exigencies of the state: An ethnomedical view. *Psychiatry, 53*, 246–261.

Fáfúnwá, B. (1969). The role of counseling and guidance in developing nations. *Careers, 1* (2), 2–7.

Feierman, S. (1985). Struggles for control: The social roots of health and healing in modern Africa. *African Studies Review*, 28, (2/3), 73–147.

Fetterman, D. M. (1989). *Ethnography, Step by step*. London: Sage.

Foster, G. M. (1976). Disease etiologies in non-Western medical systems. *American Anthropologist*, *78*, (4), 773–782.

Frank, J. D. (1961). *Persuasion and healing*. Baltimore: John Hopkins Press.

Frank, J. D. (1978). *Psychotherapy and the human predicament*. New York: Schocken.

Frey, D. H. (1978). Science and the single case in counseling research. *Personnel and Guidance Journal, 56* (5), 263–268.

Furnham, A. (1994). Explaining health and illness: Lay beliefs on the nature of health. *Personality and Individual Differences, 17* (4), 455–466.

Furnham, A. (1994). Explaining health and illness: Lay perceptions on current and future health, the causes of illness, and the nature of recovery. *Social Science and Medicine, 39* (5), 715–725.

Furnham, A. & Forey, J. (1994). The attitudes, behaviors and beliefs of patients of conventional vs complementary (alternative) medicine. *Journal of Clinical Psychology, 50* (3), 458–469.

Gardner, G. G. (1964). The psychotherapeutic relationship. *Psychological Bulletin, 61*, 426–437.

Gay, D. (1993). *Disease in Lesotho: Perception and prevalence*. A report prepared for the World Health Organization and the Ministry of Health, Government of Lesotho, under the sponsorship of the European Community.

Gay, J. & Gill, D. (1993). *Health in Lesotho: A development profile*. A report prepared for the World Health Organization and the Ministry of Health, Government of Lesotho, under the sponsorship of the European Community.

Gellert, G. (1994). Global explanations and the credibility problem of alternative medicine. *Advances, 10* (4), 60–67.

Goldman, L. (1978). *Research methods for counselors: Practical approaches in field settings*. New York: John Wiley and Sons, Inc..

Gould, J. & Kolb, W.L. (1964). *A dictionary of the social sciences*. New York: The Free Press.

Green, E. C. (1985). Traditional healers, mothers and childhood diarrheal disease in Swaziland: The interface of anthropology and health education. *Social Science and Medicine, 20* (3), 277–285.

Green, E. C., & Makhubu, L. (1984). Traditional healers in Swaziland: Toward improved cooperation between the traditional and modern health sectors. *Social Science and Medicine, 18* (12), 1071–1079.

Green, E. C. (1992). Sexually transmitted diseases, ethnomedicine and health policy in Africa. *Social Science and Medicine, 35* (2), 121–130.

Guba, E. G., & Lincoln, Y. S. (1981). *Effective evaluation: Improving the usefulness of evaluation results through responsive and naturalistic approaches*. San Francisco: Jossey Bass.

Haupt, A. (1995). *The population reference bureau's population hand book*. Washington D.C.: Population Reference Bureau.

Healers offer unique brand psychotherapy (1967). *Medical World News*, September 29.

Hickson, J. & Makhobo, D. (1992). Combating AIDS in Africa: Cultural barriers to effective prevention and treatment. *Journal of Multicultural Counseling and Development*, *20* (1), 11–22.

Hoebel, E. A. (1972). *Anthropology: The study of man*. New York: McGraw Hill Book Company.

Hughes, T. (1968). *The iron man*. London: Faber Publishing Press.

Ìdòwú, E. Bólájí (1962). *Olódùmarè: God in Yorùbá belief*. London: Longman.

Ìdòwú, A. I. (1985). Counseling Nigerian students in United States colleges and universities. *Journal of Counseling and Development*, *63*, 506–509.

Ìdòwú, A.I. (1985). Myths and superstitions in traditional healing. *American Mental Health Counselors' Association Journal*, *7* (2), 78–86.

Ìpàyẹ́, B. (1986). Roles and functions of counselors in Nigerian schools. *Nigerian Journal of Guidance and Counseling*, *2* (1), 87–106.

Ityavyar, D. A. (1987). Background to the development of health services in Nigeria. *Social Science and Medicine*, *24* (6), 487–499.

Jackson, B. (1987). *Fieldwork*. Urbana: University of Illinois Press.

Jaeger, R. M. (1988). *Complementary methods for research in education*. Washington, DC: American Educational Research Association.

Jahoda, G. (1961). Traditional healers and other institutions concerned with mental illness in Ghana. *International Journal of Social Psychiatry*, *7* (4), 245–268.

Janzen, J. M. (1992). *Ngoma: Discourses of healing in central and southern Africa*. Berkeley: University of California Press.

Johnson, J. A. (1986). *A child with a physical disability in a nuclear family: A case study*. Unpublished dissertation. George Washington University, Washington, D. C..

Kahn, M. W., & Delk, J. (1973). Developing a community mental health clinic on the Papago Indian Reservation. *International Journal of Social Psychiatry*, *19*, 299–306.

Kantor, Debra Jean (1993). Healing narratives of middle class suburban Americans (Alternative medicine). *Dissertation Abstracts*, DAI-A 54703.

Kazdin, A. E. (1980). *Research design in clinical psychology*. New York: Harper and Row Publishers.

Kelly, I. (1965). *Folk Practices in North Mexico*. Austin: University of Texas Press.

Kerlinger, Fred N. (1986). *Foundations of behavioral research* (3rd ed.). New York : Holt, Rinehart, and Winston.

Kiev, A. (1962). The psychotherapeutic aspects of primitive medicine. *Human Organization*, *21*, 25–29.

Kleinman, A. (1980). *Patients and healers in the context of culture: An exploration of the borderland between anthropology, medicine, and psychiatry*. Berkeley: University of California Press.

Kramer, B. H. (1970). Psychotherapeutic implications of a traditional healing ceremony: The Malaysian main Puteri. *Transcultural Psychiatric Research Review*, *7*,149–151.

Krippner, S. (1984). *Folk healing in Indonesia and around the world: Interview with Dr. Stanley Krippner*. San Francisco: Department of Consciousness Studies, Saybrook Institute.

Kurian, G. T. (1989). *Glossary of the Third World: words for understanding Third World peoples cultures*. New York: Facts On File.

Lámbò, T. A. (1963). *African traditional beliefs, concepts of health and medical practice*. Ìbàdàn: Ìbàdàn University Press.

Lámbò, T. A. (1969). Traditional African cultures and Western medicine in F. N. L. Poynter (ed.). *Medicine and culture*. London: Wellcome Institute of the History of Medicine.

Lámbò, T. A. (1974). Psychotherapy in Africa. *Psychotherapy and Psychosomatics*, 24, 311–326.

Lámbò, T. A. (1978). Psychotherapy in Africa. *Human Nature, 1*, 32–39. Also in *Psychotherapy and Psychosomatics (1974), 24*, 311–326.

Lámbò, T. A. (1983). Integration of traditional medicine: Another view. *Nigerian Tribune*, August 11, 2.

Lepowsky, M. (1990). Sorcery and penicillin: Treating illness on a Papua New Guinea Island. *Social Science and Medicine, 30* (10), 1049–1063.

Levers, L. L. (1996). Professional practice: Counseling as a recursive dynamic. In T. R. F. Riggar & D. R. Maki (Eds.), *Rehabilitation counseling: Profession and practice* (pp. 172–190). New York: Springer Publishing Company.

Levers, L. L. & Maki, D. R. (1995). African indigenous healing, cosmology and existential implications: Toward a philosophy of ethnorehabilitation. *Rehabilitation Education, 9* (2), 127–145.

Levers, L. L. & Maki, D. R. (1994). *An ethnographic analysis of traditional healing and rehabilitation services in Southern Africa: Crosscultural implications*. A fellowship report prepared for the World Rehabilitation Fund, National Institute on Disability and Rehabilitation Research, U. S. Department of Education, 103 pages. Oklahoma State University, Stillwater, OK: National Clearing House of Rehabilitation Training Materials.

Levine, R. A. (1973). *Culture, behavior and personality*. Chicago: Aldine.

Levine, E. S., & Padilla, A. M. (1980). *Cross cultures in therapy: Pluralistic counseling for the Hispanics*. Monterey: Brooks/Cole.

Loeb, E. (1929). Shaman and seer. *American Anthropologist, 31*, 61–84.

Mábògùnjẹ́, A. L. (1962). *Yorùbá towns: Problems of a pre-industrialized urbanization in West Africa*. Ìbàdàn: Nigeria, Ìbàdàn University Press.

MacLachlan, M. (1993). Mental health in Malawi: Which way forward? *Journal of Mental Health-UK*, 2(3), 271–274.

Mákindé, M. A. (1983). Ifá as a repository of knowledge. Paper presented at the XVIIth World Congress of Philosophy, Montreal Canada, August 21–27. Also in *Odù* (1983). *A Journal of West African Studies, 23*, 116–121.

Mákindé, M. A. (1987). Cultural and philosophical dimensions of neuro-medical sciences. *Nigerian Journal of Psychiatry*, September, 85–100.

Mákindé, M. A. (1988). *African Philosophy, culture and traditional medicine*. Athens: Ohio University Center for International Studies. Monograms in International Studies.

Mákindé, M. A. (1994). Report on, and assessment of, field work on "*Analysis of interpersonal techniques used by Yorùbá Traditional Healers of Nigeria : A case study.*" November.

Mákindé, O. (1973). *Guidance and counseling in Western Nigerian high schools utilizing the indigenous approach with the addition of Western approaches*. Unpublished doctoral dissertation. Amherst: University of Massachusetts, May.

Mákindé, O. (1974). The indigenous Babaláwo model—Implications for counseling in West Africa. *West African Journal of Education, 18* (4), 319–27.

Mákindé, O. (1976). Historical foundations of counseling in Africa. *Journal of Negro Education, XLVI* (3), 303–317.

Mákindé, O. (1980). *A survey of counseling approaches*. Paper presented at a workshop. University of Ìbàdàn, Nigeria. September 8th -12th.

Mákindé, O. (1984). *Fundamentals of guidance and counseling*. London: Macmillan.

Mallum, M. P. (1983). *Traditional helping process in Nigerian society*. The Hague, Netherlands: Martinus Nijhoff.

Mallum, M. P. (1983). Traditional helping processes in Nigerian society. *International Journal for the Advancement of Counseling, 6* (4), 289–295.

Mar'i, S. K. (1982). Cultural and socio-political influences on counseling and career guidance: The case of Arabs in the Jewish state. *International Journal for the Advancement of Counseling, 5*, 247–263.

Mbiti, J. S. (1988). *African religions and philosophy*. London: Heinemann.

McAuliffe, K. (1992). What the witchdoctor knew. *Good Housekeeping*, 214, p.1564.

McClain, C. S. (Ed.). (1989). *Women as healers: Cross-cultural perspectives*. New Brunswick: The Rutgers University Press.

McElroy, A. & Townsend, P. K. (1985). *Medical anthropology in ecological perspective*. Boulder, CO: Westview Press.

McKee, L. (1987). Ethnomedical treatment of children's diarrheal illnesses in the highlands of Ecuador. *Social Science and Medicine, 25* (10), 1147–1155.

Mead, M. (1939). *From the south seas*. New York: William Morrow.

Mead, M. (1955). *Cultural patterns and technical change*. New York: New American Library.

Mead, M. (1970). *Culture and commitment*. New York: National History Press.

Merriam, S. B. (1988). *Case study research in education*. San Francisco: Jossey Bass.

Miller, E. & Warner, R. W., Jr. (1975). Single research and evaluation. *Personnel and Guidance Journal*, November, 130–133.

Morris, B. (1986). Herbalism and divination in Southern Malawi. *Social Science and Medicine, 23* (4), 367–377.

Murphy, J. T. (1980). *Getting the facts: A fieldwork guide for evaluators and policy analysts*. Santa Monica, CA: Goodyear Publishing Company, Inc..

Murray, J. & Shepherd, S. (1993). Alternative or additional medicine? An exploratory study in general practice. *Social Science and Medicine, 37* (8), 983–988.

National Policy on Education (1981). Federal Republic of Nigeria. Lagos: Printing Division, Federal Ministry of Information.

N'donazi, B. (1991). Proving the worth of a healing art. *Time*, 138, p. 52.

Ngokwey, N. (1988). Pluralistic etiological systems in their social context: A Brazilian case study. *Social Science and Medicine, 26* (8), 793–802.

Nongu, V. A. (1984). *Traditional counseling among Tiv People of Benue State*. Unpublished masters' thesis. University of Jos, Jos, Nigeria.

Nyamwaya, D. (1987). A case study of the interaction between indigenous and Western medicine among the Pokot of Kenya. *Social Science and Medicine, 25*(12), 1277–1287.

Odẹ́bíyì, A. I. & Togonu-Bickersteth, F. (1987). Concepts and management of deafness in the Yorùbá medical system: A case study of traditional healers in Ilé-Ifẹ̀, Nigeria. *Social Science and Medicine, 24* (8), 645–649.

Ọdẹ́bíyì, A. I. (1989). Food taboos in maternal and child health: The view of traditional healers in Ilé-Ifẹ̀, Nigeria. *Social Science and Medicine, 27* (9), 985–996.

Ọdẹ́jídé, O. A., Ohaeri, J. U., Adélẹ̀kàn, M. L., & Ikúesan, B. A. (1989). Alcohol treatment systems in Nigeria. *Alcohol and Alcoholism, 24* (4), 347–353.

Ọdẹ́jídé, A. O., Ọlátawúrà, M. O., Sàndà, A. O., & Oyènẹ́yẹ, A. O. (1977). Traditional Healers and mental illness in the city of Ìbàdàn. *African Journal of Psychiatry, 3*, 99–106.

Òjó, G. J. (1967). *Yorùbá culture*. London: University of Ifẹ̀ and University of London Press.

Okon, S. (1983). Guidance and counseling services in Nigeria. *Personnel and Guidance Journal, 61*, (8), 457–459.

Ọláyínká, M. S. (1973). *Counselor preparation and his functions in the Nigerian educational system*. Seminar paper on Lagos counseling and guidance. Child Guidance Clinic, Yábà. November.

Ọláyínká, M. S. (1976). The place of counseling in Nigerian educational policy. *Nigerian Journal of Psychology, 1*, 89–93.

Oyèbọ̀lá, D. D. O. (1980). The method of training traditional healers and midwives among the Yorùbá of Nigeria. *Social Science and Medicine, 14A*, 31–37.

Oyèbọ̀lá, D. D. O. (1980). Traditional medicine and its practitioners among the Yorùbá of Nigeria: A classification. *Social Science and Medicine, 14A*, 23–29.

Ozekhome, F. E. A. (1992). *The theory and practice of traditional medicine in Nigeria*. Lagos, Nigeria: Okey Okwechime.

Pedersen, P. (1983). The cultural complexity of counseling. *International Journal for the Advancement of Counseling*, 6, 177–192.

Pedersen, D., & Coloma, C. (1983). Traditional medicine in Ecuador: The structure of the non-formal health systems. *Social Science and Medicine, 17*(17), 1249–1255.

Pedersen, A., & Pedersen, P. (1989). The cultural grid: A framework for multicultural counseling. *International Journal for the Advancement of Counseling, 12*, 299–307.

Peters, L. G. (1981). An experiential study of Nepalese Shamanism. *The Journal of Transpersonal Psychology*, 13, (1), 4–23.

Pierre, H. (1969). Western medicine and Afro-American ethnic medicine in F. N. L. Poynter (Ed.), *Medicine and culture*. London: Welcome Institute of the History of Medicine, New Series, Volume XV, 211–237.

Prince, R. (1962). *Some notes on Yorùbá native doctors and their management of mental illness*. In T. A. Lámbò (Ed.), First Pan African Psychiatric Conference. Ìbàdàn, Nigeria: Government Printer.

Prince, R. (1964). Indigenous Yorùbá psychiatry. In A. Kiev (Ed.), *Magic, faith and healing*. New York: The Free Press.

Prince, R. (1976). Psychotherapy as the manipulation of indigenous healing mechanisms: A transcultural survey. *Transcultural Psychiatric Research Review, 13*, 115–133.

Punch, M. (1986). *The politics and ethics of fieldwork*. Beverly Hills: Sage.

Qidraogo, A. J. (1989). The old and the new. *World Health*, March, 23–24.

Rankin, S. B. & Kappy, M. S. (1993). Developing therapeutic relationships in multicultural settings. *Academic Medicine, 68* (11), 826–827.

Rappaport, H. (1977). The tenacity of folk psychotherapy: A functional interpretation. *Social Psychiatry, 12 (3)*, 127–132.

Roder, W. (1991). Magic, medicine and metaphysics in Nigeria. *Skeptical Inquirer, 15*, 290–295.

Salan, R., & Maretzki, T. (1983). Mental health services and traditional healing in Indonesia: Are the roles compatible? *Culture, Medicine and Psychiatry*, 7 (4), 377–412.

Saleh, M. (1986). Cultural perspectives: Implications for counseling in the Arab world. *International Journal of School Psychology*, 7 (2), 10–17.

Saleh, M. A. (1989). The cultural milieu of counseling. *International Journal for the Advancement of Counseling,* 12, 3–11.

Sàndà, A. O. (1978). The scientific or magical ways of knowing: Implications for the study of African Traditional healers. *Second Order, VII*, (1&2), January and July, 70–83.

Schoepf, B.G. (1992). AIDS, sex and condoms: African healers and the reinvention of tradition in Zaire. Special issue: Rethinking AIDS prevention. *Medical Anthropology, 14* (2–4), 225–242.

Schusky, E. L., & Culbert, T. P. (1967). *Introduction to culture*. Englewood Cliffs, NJ: Prentice Hall.

Sherman, H. (1967). *"Wonder" healers of the Philippines*. Los Angeles, CA: DeVorss.

Singer, M. (1984). Spiritual healing and family therapy: Common approaches to the treatment of alcoholism. *Family Therapy, XI* (2), 155–162.

Smith, R. B. (1982). *An introduction to social research (Vol 1): Handbook of social science methods*. Cambridge, MA: Ballinger.

Ṣófowórà, A. (1981). *Man, plants and medicine in Africa*. An inaugural lecture delivered at the University of Ifẹ̀, Nigeria, January 7.

Stoller, P. (1989). *Fusion of the worlds: An ethnography of possession among the Songhay of Niger*. Chicago: University of Chicago Press.

Sundberg, N. S. (1977). *Assessment of persons*. New Jersey: Prentice Hall.

Torrey, E. F. (1969). The case for the indigenous therapist. *Archives of General Psychiatry, 20*, 365–373.

Torrey, E. F. (1972). *The mind game: Witch doctors and psychiatrists*. New York: Emerson Hall.

Torrey, E. F. (1980). Traditional medical practitioners: Pros and cons. *Lancet, 1*, 963–964.

Torrey, E. F. (1986). *Witch doctors and psychiatrists: The common roots of psychotherapy and its future*. New York: Harper and Row.

The Traditional background to medical practice in Nigeria (1966) & (1981). Occasional Publication, University of Ìbàdàn, Nigeria: Institute of African Studies in Collaboration with Ìbàdàn University College Hospital April 20–23.

Trachtman, P. (1994). National Institute of Health (NIH) looks at the implausible and the inexplicable. *Smithsonian, 25* (6), 110–123.

Tylor, E. (1989). *The primitive culture*. New York: Henry Holt & Co..

Umoren, U. E. (1990). Religion and traditional medicine: An anthropological case study of a Nigerian treatment of mental illness. *Medical Anthropology, 12* (4), 389–400.
UNICEF—WHO (1975). Joint committee on health policy report of the 20th session held at the headquarters of *World Health Organization, Geneva*, 4–6, February.
Van Dalen, D. B. & Meyer, W. J.(1966). *Understanding educational research: An introduction*. New York: McGraw Hill.
van Manen, M. (1990). *Researching lived experience: Human science for an action sensitive pedagogy*. New York: State University of New York Press.
Veyrat, J. G. & Ferrier J. (1989). From Haiti voodoo and Brazilian candomble to European hypernea: Applications to psychosomatic medicine. *Annales Medico Psychologigues*, *147* (3), 341–347.
Vontress, C. E. (1991). Traditional healing in Africa: Implications for cross-cultural counseling. *Journal of Counseling and Development*, *70* (1), 242–249.
Waldram, J.B. (1990). Access to traditional medicine in a western Canadian city. *Medical Anthropology, 12* (3), 325–348.
Wallace, A. F. C. (1970). *Culture and personality* (2nd ed.). New York: Random House.
Watson, R. I. (1963). *The clinical method in psychology*. New York: Harper and Brothers Publications.
Weiss, M.G. et al. (1986). Traditional concepts of mental disorder among Indian psychiatric patients: Preliminary report of work in progress. *Social Science and Medicine*, *23* (4), 379–386.
Witmer, M. L. & Sweeney, T. J. (1992). A holistic model for wellness and prevention over the life span. *Journal of Counseling and Development, 71*, 140–148.
Witte, K. (1991). The role of culture in health and disease. In L. Samovar & R. Porter (Eds.), *Intercultural Communication: A reader* (6th ed.). Belmont, CA: Wadsworth, 199–206.
The World Almanac and book of facts (1995). New Jersey: Funk and Wagnalls Corporation, 806–807.
World Health Organization. (1975). *Training and utilization of traditional healers and their collaboration with Health Care delivery systems*. Provisional Agenda, item 17, No. EB 57/21 226, 53; add 2. Fifty-seventh Session of the Executive Board. Geneva: May.
World Health Organization (1976). African Traditional Medicine. *Afro Technical Report Series, No 1*. Congo Brazaville: WHO Regional Office for Africa.
World Health Organization. (1978). *Primary Health Care: Report of the International Conference on Primary Health Care*. Alma-Ata: United Soviet Socialist Republics (USSR). Geneva.
World Health Organization (1978). The promotion and development of traditional medicine. *W.H.O. Technical Report Series, 622*, 1–41. Geneva.
Yin, R. K. (1984). *Case study research: Design and methods*. Newbury Park, CA: Sage.
Yin, R. K. (1994). *Case study research: Design and methods*. Thousand Oaks, CA: Sage.

Appendix A

Discussions of the Taped Conversation between Chief Àràbà of Ilé-Ifẹ̀, the profiled Chief Diviner and Professor Michael Akin Mákindé, the Researcher's Consultant on November 20, 1994.

The purpose of the discussion was to enlighten the researcher on the roles of ***Oníṣègùn*** **(Herbalists)** and ***Ifá priests*** **(Diviners)** in *Yorùbá* traditional counseling and medicine. Herbalists are Yorùbá Traditional Healers who mix, dispense and cure diseases with herbs, and also counsel clients who have problems. Diviners are Yorùbá Traditional Healers who use divining chains and beads to consult *Ifá oracle* about the sources of clients' illnesses, diseases and problems.

1. Differences between Diviners and Herbalists

Herbalists sometimes depend on diviners who, through *Ifá*, know the right herbs needed for treatment. Some herbalists may find it difficult to treat patients unless they consult *Ifá* oracle to inquire about what obstacles are likely to impede effective treatment and cure. Thus, it is usually said that evil forces must be eliminated before success could be attained in the treatment of certain ailments, which cannot be treated by orthodox medical practitioners. Therefore, Chief Àràbà specified that, ***"kí a mú ti èṣù kúrò."*** (Let us remove the enemy's hand from the problems at hand).

Chief Àràbà agrees with Professor Michael Mákindé, the researcher's consultant, that **herbalists** are very powerful practitioners that **diviners** need, and that both of them complement each other's efforts.

2. Yorùbá Traditional Counseling

The method of counseling by ***Ifá*** **priests** is different from the ***Oníṣègùns***. By virtue of his oracular power, the ***Ifá*** **priest** comes to know the problem of his client divining using the *Ifá* oracle. It is from this point of view that the ***babaláwo*** begins to counsel his client and advise him on what to do, how to do it, and when to do it. He does not expect the client to disregard his advice and counseling, as he sometimes warns the client about the consequences of not cooperating with him. The question of lying or faking an issue or complaint does not arise, since *Ifá* says what is presented before it. So if there is a problem *Ifá* says so; if there is none it says so as well.

On the other hand, the ***Oníṣègùn*** has no means of finding out his client's problem unless the client tells him or examines him or her. He depends on observation, which is, observing the client and questioning her or him or his or her relatives about some antecedent events. For example, questions regarding when a client or patient was born, what led to his or her sickness, and how and when the sickness started are asked. ***Ifá* priests** sometimes advise clients against doing certain things because of the consequences. It is generally agreed among the ***Yorùbá*** that, ***Ọ̀rúnmìlà*** is the owner of *Ifá* while, ***Ọ̀sanyìn***, ***Ọ̀rúnmìlà's*** servant, is the father and initiator of herbal knowledge and medicine.

Appendix B
Interview Schedule

Interview Schedule

Yorùbá questions used to elicit information from five Yorùbá Traditional Healers: four Herbalists and one Diviner, interviewed in Ọ̀yọ́, Ọ̀sun, Ọ̀gùn, and Ondò states of Nigeria.

YORÙBÁ SCRIPT

ÀWỌN ÌBÉÈRÈ FÚN ÀWỌN BABALÁWO MÉJE: ONÍṢÈGÙN MẸRIN ÀTI ALAFOSE KAN TÍ MO FI ẸRỌ ÌYANILÁWÒRÁN ÀTI ERO ÌGBA OHÙN SÌLẸ̀ BÁ SỌ̀RỌ̀.

Ẹ kú àárọ Bàbá wa.

Mo wá sí ọ̀dọ̀ yín láti fi ẹ̀rọ yìí ya àwòrán irú ìjíròrò tí ó máa n lọ láàárín ẹ̀yin àti àwọn tí wọ́n n wá sí ọ̀dọ̀ yín ní gbogbo ìgbà. N ó sì fi ẹ̀rọ ìgba ohùn sílẹ̀ yìí gba àwọn ọ̀rọ̀ tí ẹ bá sọ sílẹ̀ pẹ̀lú.

Àwọn ọ̀gá mi láti ibi tí mo ti n kọ́ iṣẹ́ fún àti máa ran àwọn onírúurú ènìyàn lọ́wọ́ ni wọ́n gbà mí nímọ̀ràn láti lọ ṣe ìfi ọ̀rọ̀ wá ni lẹ́nuwò yìí. Inú mi dùn nígbà ti wọ́n dárúkọ yín gẹ́gẹ́ bí enìkan pàtàkì tí ó ti ran ọ̀gọ̀rọ̀ ènìyàn lọ́wọ́, tí ó sì tún sì n ràn wọ́n lọ́ wọ́ síbẹ́.

Mo sì mọ̀ pé mo ṣe orí ire lónìí láti lè ṣe àkíyèsí bí iṣẹ́ yín ti fi ìdí múlẹ̀ di àsìkò yìí.

Láì fi àsìkò ṣòfò mo fẹ́ kí ẹ gba ẹ̀bùn kékeré yìí fún ànfàní tí ẹ fún èmi ọmọ yín láti ṣe ìfi ọ̀rọ̀ wáni lẹ̀nu wò yìí. Ẹ má bínú pé ó kéré. Ní agbára lọ́wọ́ Ọlọ́run tí mo bá kó ẹsẹ̀ járí nínú ẹ̀kọ́ mi èmi ó lè ra nnkan tí ó tóbi ju eléyìí lọ wá fún nyín. Lẹ́ẹ̀kan si, mo dúpẹ́ púpọ̀ fún ànfàni tí ẹ fún mi yìí. Ọlọ́run á ṣe ẹ̀yín àti àwọn ẹbí yín ní olóríire, Àmín. Ọmọ áti ọmọ dé ọmọ yín náà yóò ṣe orí ire o, Àmín. Àwọn náà yóò sì gbé igbá orókè, Àmín.

Ohun tí n ó kọ́kọ́ ṣe ni, bíbèèrè bí ẹ ṣe bẹ̀rẹ̀ iṣẹ́ yìí lọ́wọ́ yín. Lẹ́yìn náà, n ó wá lo ẹ̀rọ amóhùn máwòrán yìí láti ya bí ẹ ṣe máa n káràmásìkí àwọn tí ó n wá sí ọ̀dọ̀ yín lójojúmọ, tí ó nmú wọn padà wá fún oríṣirísi ìbéèrè àti ọ̀rọ̀ ìṣírí fún ìgbé ayé wọn ní àsìkò dé àsìkò. N ó yà àwòrán yìí ní ẹ̀ẹ̀marùn-ún, fún ìgbà kọ̀ọ̀kan tí ẹ bá rí abẹ̀wé ọkùnrin tàbí obìnrin kọ̀ọ̀kan tí ó bá wá sí ọ́dọ́ yín. Ẹ̀yì ni yóò fún mi láyè láti rí **ìṣesí** yín àti ìwà yín tí ó ngbé yín lárugẹ lójú àwọn abẹ̀wé.

ÌBÉÈRÈ

(I) Ìpín ìkìnní: Ìbí yín
1. Níbo ni a bí yín sí?
2. Àsìkò wo ni a bí yín?
3. Ọdún wo ni a bí yín?
4. Ọmọ ọdún mélòó ni yín?
5. Nnkan pàtàkì wo ni ó ṣẹlẹ̀ nígbà tí a bí yín tí ó fún àwọn òbí yín ní ààmì pé irú iṣẹ́ yìí ni ẹ ó ṣe?
6. Ṣé ibi tí a bí yín sí nì yíí?
7. Ṣé ibòmíràn ni ẹ ti wà síbí láti wá ṣiṣẹ́ yìí?
8. Ìwé òyìnbó mélòó ni ẹ kà?

(II) **Ìpín èkejì: Iṣẹ́ yín**
1. Ìgbà wo ni ẹ bẹ̀rẹ̀ iṣẹ́ yìí?
2. Báwo ni ẹ ṣe bẹ̀rẹ̀ iṣẹ́ yìí?
3. Ibo ni ẹ ti gba agbára tàbí àṣẹ láti máa ṣe iṣẹ́ yìí?
   (a) àjogúnbá?
   (b) àti ọ̀dọ̀ Ọlọ́run?
   (d) àti ọ̀dọ̀ àwọn àgbà tí ó kọ́ yín ní iṣẹ́?
   (e) àti ojú àlá?
   (f) ibòmirán? (**ṣe àpèjúwe**)
4. Ọdún mélòó ni ẹ lò ní ẹnu ẹ̀kọṣẹ́ kí ẹ tó bẹ̀rẹ̀ iṣẹ́ yìí?
5. Ta ni ó kọ yín ní iṣẹ́ yìí?
6. Ṣé ẹ tún n ṣe iṣẹ́ miràn mọ́ iṣẹ́ yìí?
7. Ènìyàn mélòó ni ó mọ̀ yín lẹ́nu iṣẹ́ yìí?
8. Ẹ jọ̀wọ̀ ẹ ṣe àpèjúwe ibi tí òkìkí yín ti tàn dé ní ẹnu iṣẹ́ yìí?

(III) **Ìpín Ìkẹta:** Irú ènìyàn tí wọn jẹ
1. Ìyàwó mélòó ni ẹ ní?
2. Ṣé ìyàwó yín fẹ́ràn iṣẹ́ yín?
3. Ṣé ìyàwó yín n bá yín ṣẹ́ iṣẹ́ yìí?
4. Ọmọ mélòó ni ẹ bí?
5. Àbúrò mélòó ni ẹ ní?
6. Mélòó nínú àwọn ọmọ yín ni ó n ṣe iṣẹ́ yìí?
7. Mélòó nínú àwọn ọmọ yín ló wà lẹ́nu ìkọ́ṣe lọ́dọ́ yín tàbí lọ́dọ́ ẹ̀lòmíràn ní lóólóó yìí?
8. Mélòó nínú àwọn ọmọ yín ni ó máa kọ́ iṣẹ́ yìí ní ọjọ́ iwájú?

9. Ipò kelóò ni ẹ jẹ́ nínú ọmọ bábà yín?
10. Kí ni irú iṣẹ́ tí bàbá yín fún yín ṣe gẹ́gẹ́ bí olú ọmọ nígbà tí ẹ kéré?
11. Ṣé nnkan mìràn wà tí ẹ fẹ́ sọ fún mi nípa ara yín nígbà tí ẹ kéré tàbí nígbà tí ẹ dàgbà tí mi ò rántí láti bèèrè tí yóò ràn mí lọ́wọ́ láti mọ ìdí tí ẹ fi ní òkìkì ní ẹnu iṣẹ́ yín?

(IV)Ìpín èkẹrin: Ìríri Ayé (Experience)

1. Ẹ jọ̀wọ́ ẹ sọ ìrírí yín nípa ayé ní sókí gẹ́gẹ́ bí oníṣègùn pàtàkì tí ó lókìkí lẹnu iṣẹ́ yìí?

(V) Ìpín Ìkarùn-ún: Ìṣesí yín sí àwọn ènìyàn tí ó nwá sí ọ̀dọ̀ yín (Interactions)

1. Báwo ni ìṣesí yín sí àwọn abewé tí wọn n wá sí ọ̀dọ̀ yín? (**behavior**)
2. Kí ni èrò ọkàn yín sí àwọn abewé tí wọ́n bá wá sí ọ̀dọ̀ yín? (**feelings**)
3. Kí ni ètò tí ẹ máa n ṣe pẹ̀lú àwọn abewé tí wọ́n bá wá sí ọ̀dọ̀ yín? (**plan**)
4. Kí ni ètò tí ẹ máa n ṣe pẹ̀lú àwọn abewé nípa ohun tí ó wù kí wọ́n bá wá sí ọdọ yín? (**plan**)
5. Báwo ni ẹ ṣe n ṣe sí áwọn abewé ní gbogbo ìgbà tí wọ́n bá wá sí ọdọ yín? (**attitude**)
6. Ànfàní wo ni àwọn abewé n rí gbà lọ́dọ́ yín tí ẹ rò pé ó n mú wọn padà wá lójojúmọ́ fún ìrànlọ́wọ́ lọ́dọ́ yín?
7. Kí ni èrò ọkàn yín láti jẹ́ kí iṣẹ́ yín máa lọ déédéé?
8. Kí ni ọkàn yín máa n fẹ́ ṣe sí àwọ̀n abewé nígbà tí wọ́n bá wá sí ọ́dọ́ yín fún ìjíròrò tàbí fún ìṣòro kíṣòro?
9. Kí ni ọkàn yín máa n fẹ́ ṣe sí àwọn abewé nígbà tí ẹ bá n bá wọn jíròrò nípa ohun tí ó wù kí wọ́n bá wá?
10. Kí ni ohun mìràn tí ẹ fẹ́ kí n mọ̀ nípa iṣe yín sí àwọn abewé tí wọ́n n wá sí ọ̀dọ̀ yín tí í ṣe ìṣínilórí fún wọn láti padà wá nígbà gbogbo?
11. Irú ìlànà wo ni ẹ máa n lò pẹ̀lú àwọn abewé tí wọ́n nwá sí ọdọ yín fún àmọ̀ràn tàbí fún ìwòsàn?
12. Kí ni ohun miràn tí ẹ fẹ́ kí n mò nípa bí ẹ ti n ṣe iṣẹ́ yìí tí n kò rántí bèrè? Ẹ ṣe púpọ̀ fún fífi àsìkò sílẹ̀ fún mi láti ṣe ìjíròrò yìí pẹ̀lú yín. Ọlọ́run Olódùmarè á jẹ́ kí ẹ pẹ fún wa o. Àmín. A ó máa rí yín bá o. Ámín.

Appendix C
Interview Schedule

English language translations of Yorùbá questions used to elicit information from five Yorùbá Traditional Healers: four Herbalists (Onísègùn) and one Diviner (Ifá Priest), interviewed in Òyó, Òsun, Ògùn, and Ondò states of Nigeria.

ENGLISH LANGUAGE TRANSLATION

Good morning, our fathers.

I have come to you this morning to use this videotape equipment to capture the interactions that take place between you and the clients who come to you for counseling.

My advisers at my university, where I am learning how to counsel individuals, encouraged me to come and inquire about your sources of expertise from you. I was happy when your name was mentioned as one important personality in the community who has been of assistance and who still continues to be of assistance to numerous clients. I know that I am opportuned to be able to come and observe how your interactions with clients have been excellently renowned to be of good reputation/foundation until now. Without wasting much time, I am presenting this gift to you for giving me the opportunity to ask questions and to observe your interactions with your clients.

Thank you for giving me this opportunity. I promise to show further gratitude when I finish my academic endeavors. My prayer is that you and all the members of your family excel and succeed in all your undertakings. Amen.

The first set of questions will focus on how you started your healing work. After this set of questions, I will videotape the modes of interaction between you and the clients who come to you for help in your clinic. I intend to videotape one interaction each for five clients who visit you. The video-taped session will allow me to observe your interactions with your clients, and to perceive how this mode of interaction has encouraged clients to continue to patronize you.

QUESTIONS

Section I: Birth

1. Where were you born?
2. What time were you born?
3. What year were you born?
4. How old are you?
5. What important thing happened at your birth to show your parents that you were set apart to be a traditional healer?
6. Were you born in this town?
7. Were you brought from another place to work here as a healer?
8. What grade level of Western education did you finish?

Section II: Work Setting

1. When did you start this work?
2. How did you start this work?
3. How did you obtain the power, or authority to start this work, through:
   (a) Inheritance
   (b) From God Almighty (*Olódùmarè*)
   (c) From elders who trained you to master this work.
   (d) From dreams/dream invoked
   (e) Other sources not mentioned above
   (please describe)
4. How many years of apprenticeship did you spend learning this work before you graduated?
5. Who taught you this work?
6. Do you perform other duties/work in addition to divining/healing?
7. How many individuals know you in this work?
8. How far does your fame extend in this work?

Section III: Personality

1. How many wives do you have?
2. Does your wife (wives) assist you in doing this work?
3. How many children do you have?
4. How many siblings do you have?
5. How many of your children do this work with you?
6. How many of your children are presently learning this work under your supervision or somebody else's supervision?

7. How many of your children will learn this work in the near future?
8. What is your birth position among your father's children?
9. What type of work did your father give you as a special child when you were growing up?
10. Please explain any other information that I forgot to ask that will prove useful in explaining the reasons for your fame and popularity in this work.

SECTION IV: EXPERIENCE IN THE WORLD

1. Please explain briefly your experience in this work as a well-known traditional healer (diviner or herbalist).

SECTION V: INTERACTIONS WITH CLIENTS

1. How do you behave to clients who consult you?
2. What do you think and feel towards your clients when they consult you?
3. What plan do you have for your clients when they come to you for healing?
4. What plan do you have for your clients in terms of the unique problems that they bring to you?
5. What are your attitudes toward your clients when they come to you for counseling and healing?
6. What advantages do you think clients derive from you that encourage them to come back or recommend someone else to you?
7. What are your plans for making your work with clients progress for the better?
8. What plans do you conceive toward your clients when they consult you for their different problems?
9. What are your thoughts toward your clients as you assist them with their problems?
10. What other explanations can you give me in addition to the above that encourages clients to consult you, and which also makes you renowned among them?
11. What techniques do you use with your clients who come to you for counseling or healing?
12. What other points can you add to the above that I have forgotten to ask you?

Thank very much for your time. May you live long for us to continue to consult with. Amen.

Tables

Table 1. Healer Characteristics

Demographic Variable	Herbalist 1	Herbalist 2	Herbalist 3	Herbalist 4	Chief Diviner
Age	73	62	84	85	62
Education	No Formal Western Education	Chartered Accountant	No Formal Western Education	College Graduate	No Formal Western Education
Family					
Married	Yes	Yes	Yes	Yes	Yes
Wives	Many	1	Many	Many	Many
Children	Many	7	Many	Many	Many
Siblings	Many	Many	Many	Many	Many
Years Experenced	47 Years	30 Years	52 Years	68 Years	22 Years
Religion	Christian	Muslim	Traditional	Christian	Traditional
Sources of Power					
*apprenticeship	Yes	Yes	Yes	Yes	Yes
* observations	Yes	Yes	Yes	Yes	Yes
* natural endowment	Yes				
* self-teaching			Yes	Yes	Yes
* genetic dispositions	Yes	Yes			
* dreams			Yes	Yes	Yes
* close meetings and associations with :					
* god almighty (*olódùmarè*)	Yes	Yes			
* the gods	No	Yes	Yes	Yes	Yes
* ancestors	Yes	Yes	Yes	Yes	Yes
* supernatural beings	Yes	Yes			
* others	Also Fasts and Offers Prayers to Olódùmarè	Offers Prayers Five Times a Day to Allah Endowed with the Spirit of Discernment	Consults with Diviners and Other Healers on How to Assist Clients		Also Taught by Supernatural Beings

Table 2. Healer Support for Hypothesis

Hypo #s	Healer 1	Healer 2	Healer 3	Healer 4	Healer 5	Healer 6	Healer 7
1.							
Sources of Power							
apprenticeship	Yes	Yes	Yes	Yes	No	Yes	Yes
observations	Yes	Yes	Yes	Yes	No	Yes	Yes
natural endowment	Yes	Yes	Yes	Yes	Yes	Yes	Yes
self-teaching	Yes	Yes	Yes	Yes	Yes	Yes	Yes
genetic dispositions	Yes	Yes	No	Yes	Yes	Yes	Yes
dreams	Yes	Yes	Yes	Yes	Yes	Yes	Yes
close meetings with:							
God Almighty Olódùmarè	Yes	Yes	No	Yes	Yes	Yes	Yes
the gods	No	No	Yes	No	Yes	Yes	Yes
ancestors	No	Yes	Yes	No	Yes	Yes	Yes
supernatural beings	Yes	Yes	Yes	Yes	Yes	Yes	Yes
2.							
Concentrate on their clients' physical, mental, emotional, and spiritual facets during counseling and healing.	Yes	Yes	Yes	Yes	Yes	Yes	Yes
3.							
Believe that prayer to God Almighty (Olódùmare) completes healing	Yes	Yes	Yes	Yes	Yes	Yes	Yes
4.							
Use sacrifices,	Yes	Yes	Yes	Yes	Yes	Yes	Yes
divining,							
herbarium,	Yes	Yes	Yes	Yes	Yes	Yes	Yes
therapeutic dances	Yes	Yes	Yes	Yes	Yes	Yes	Yes
entreating and invoking the gods and ancestors	Yes	Yes	Yes	Yes	Yes	Yes	Yes
incision							
family supported counseling as techniques to help clients better their lives	Yes	Yes	Yes	Yes	Yes	Yes	Yes

Hypo #s	Healer 1	Healer 2	Healer 3	Healer 4	Healer 5	Healer 6	Healer 7
5.							
Consider mercy (*àánú*)	Yes	Yes	Yes	Yes	Yes	Yes	Yes
character (*ìwà*)	Yes	Yes	Yes	Yes	Yes	Yes	Yes
kindness (*inú rere*)	Yes	Yes	Yes	Yes	Yes	Yes	Yes
assistance (*ìrànlọ́wọ́*)	Yes	Yes	Yes	Yes	Yes	Yes	Yes
concern (*aájò*)	Yes	Yes	Yes	Yes	Yes	Yes	Yes
encouragement (*gbígba eni níyànjú*)	Yes	Yes	Yes	Yes	Yes	Yes	Yes
hard work (*isé àsekára*)	Yes	Yes	Yes	Yes	Yes	Yes	Yes
endurance (*ìfaradà*)	Yes	Yes	Yes	Yes	Yes	Yes	Yes
humility (*ìrẹ̀lẹ̀*)	Yes	Yes	Yes	Yes	Yes	Yes	Yes
esteeming others (*pípón ènìyàn lé*)	Yes	Yes	Yes	Yes	Yes	Yes	Yes
and patience *fífi ara balè* as basic foundations for successful healing outcomes with their clients	Yes	Yes	Yes	Yes	Yes	Yes	Yes
6.							
Use care, empathy,	Yes	Yes	Yes	Yes	Yes	Yes	Yes
respect, compassion,	Yes	Yes	Yes	Yes	Yes	Yes	Yes
patience, hard work,	Yes	Yes	Yes	Yes	Yes	Yes	Yes
consistency, faith in	Yes	Yes	Yes	Yes	Yes	Yes	Yes
God Almighty *Olódùmarè,*							
constant prayer,	Yes	Yes	Yes	Yes	Yes	Yes	Yes
a probing mind,	Yes	Yes	Yes	Yes	Yes	Yes	Yes
fear of God,	Yes	Yes	Yes	Yes	Yes	Yes	Yes
humility,	Yes	Yes	Yes	Yes	Yes	Yes	Yes
attention to details of clients', problems,	Yes	Yes	Yes	Yes	Yes	Yes	Yes
eagerness to offer services, and continual presence with their clients allow for positive therapeutic and healing outcomes	Yes	Yes	Yes	Yes	Yes	Yes	Yes
7.							
Share the same culture, experience, understanding and world view of disease, illness and problem with clients	Yes	Yes	Yes	Yes	Yes	Yes	Yes

Index

For Product Safety Concerns and Information please contact our EU representative GPSR@taylorandfrancis.com
Taylor & Francis Verlag GmbH, Kaufingerstraße 24, 80331 München, Germany

www.ingramcontent.com/pod-product-compliance
Ingram Content Group UK Ltd.
Pitfield, Milton Keynes, MK11 3LW, UK
UKHW022121190926
475702UK00013B/1566
* 9 7 8 0 4 1 5 6 5 4 8 1 4 *